Ordinary and Extraordinary
Means of Conserving Life

Ordinary and Extraordinary Means of Conserving Life

Daniel A. Cronin

❧

With a foreword by
Marie T. Hilliard

The National Catholic Bioethics Center
Philadelphia

Ordinary and Extraordinary Means of Conserving Life was first published in 1958 as Father Daniel Cronin's doctoral dissertation, under the title "The Moral Law in Regard to the Ordinary and Extraordinary Means of Conserving Life." It was later included in *Conserving Human Life*, ed. Russell E. Smith (Braintree, MA: Pope John XXIII Medical-Moral Research and Educational Center, 1989). The text has been lightly edited for the current edition, and a bibliography and index of authors have been added.

Cover design: Nicholas Furton
© 2011 The National Catholic Bioethics Center
All rights reserved
ISBN 978-0-935372-55-7

Unless otherwise noted, quotations from official Church documents are from the Vatican English translation, published online at www.vatican.va.

Library of Congress Cataloging-in-Publication Data

Cronin, Daniel Anthony, 1927-
  Ordinary and extraordinary means of conserving life / Daniel A. Cronin.
      p. cm.
  Originally presented as the author's thesis (doctoral--Gregorian University in Rome, 1958) under the title: The moral law in regard to the ordinary and extraordinary means of conserving life.
  Includes bibliographical references (p.   ) and index.
  ISBN 978-0-935372-55-7 (alk. paper)
  1. Terminal care--Moral and ethical aspects. 2. Terminal care--Religious aspects--Catholic Church. 3. Life and death, Power over--Moral and ethical aspects. 4. Life and death, Power over--Religious aspects--Catholic Church. I. Title.
  R726.C76 2011
  616.02'9--dc23
                                        2011045368

꒜

This Fiftieth Anniversary Edition is presented to
Archbishop Cronin by his friends in appreciation for
his many years of dedicated service to the Church.

MOST REVEREND MICHAEL R. COTE
Bishop of Norwich, Connecticut

EDWARD CARDINAL EGAN
Archbishop Emeritus of New York

JOHN M. HAAS
President of The National Catholic Bioethics Center
Philadelphia, Pennsylvania

MOST REVEREND WILLIAM E. LORI
Bishop of Bridgeport, Connecticut

MOST REVEREND HENRY J. MANSELL
Archbishop of Hartford, Connecticut

ST. EDMUND'S ENDERS ISLAND
Mystic, Connecticut

ST. FRANCIS HOSPITAL AND MEDICAL CENTER
Hartford, Connecticut

꒜

Contents

continued

FOREWORD

by Marie T. Hilliard

When the young Boston priest Father Daniel Cronin was directed to undertake doctoral studies in sacred theology at the Gregorian University in Rome by his Archbishop, Richard J. Cushing, he had no idea the influence his efforts would wield in the field of medical ethics over the following decades. His doctoral dissertation, defended in 1956 and published in 1958, continues to be virtually the only comprehensive historical analysis of Catholic moral teaching on ordinary and extraordinary means of conserving human life. In a letter to his dissertation director of 1954, he wrote, "I have already checked and found that the thesis has not been done at any other major university here in Europe or in America." The same statement can be made today, more than fifty years after the dissertation's original publication. The influence of the work of that young priest—now Archbishop Emeritus (Hartford)

Marie T. Hilliard, RN, PhD, JCL, is the Director of Bioethics and Public Policy at The National Catholic Bioethics Center. She worked for a number of years under Archbishop Cronin's guidance as the Executive Director of the Connecticut Catholic Conference in Hartford.

Daniel A. Cronin, STD—endures, so much so that demand favors this new edition of his now-classic work.

There have been many medical advances and challenges since 1958. At the time of the dissertation, organ transplantation was in its infancy, the first successful transplant having been performed in in 1954. Health care reimbursement mechanisms that affect the allocation of resources, such as managed care contracting, had not yet been developed. Most importantly, society had not embraced the relativism of situation ethics. Yet as these trends continue to shape society, one consistent ethic has been guarded and elucidated by the Catholic Church since its earliest days, namely, that of the natural moral law. Cronin's dissertation provides a beacon of this light of truth as it has endured throughout the centuries.

Cronin identifies and applies Church teaching to medical treatment from the thirteenth century to the middle of the twentieth century. At each point in history, advances in medicine, with case-specific examples, are analyzed in relationship to the obligation to conserve life. Cronin shows how, centuries before society was faced with questions like those raised by the case of Terri Schiavo, theological insight into a set of consistently recognized obligations to conserve life has provided both physician and patient with moral direction. That same tradition also identifies a relative norm under which these imperatives would not be considered obligatory. Theological distinctions across the centuries cross the various categories of illnesses (terminal, chronic, and life threatening) and their related obligations, especially as those obligations pertain to the common good. Of particular importance is Cronin's coverage of patient and patient-surrogate consent, even to extraordinary means—consent that often imposes an obligation on the physician to provide treatment. This obligation still holds, as described in the *Ethical and Religious Directives for Catholic Health Care*

Services (2009), unless a therapeutic intervention is contrary to Catholic principles or likely to cause harm that is disproportionate to patient benefit.

Cronin's dissertation predates the first papal teaching on ordinary and extraordinary means. It was not until November 24, 1957, that Pope Pius XII, in his landmark address to an international congress of anesthesiologists, elucidated such distinctions, particularly on questions of resuscitative measures. No papal documents before or since contradict Cronin's work. Clarifications have been provided, for example, from the Congregation for the Doctrine of the Faith on assisted nutrition and hydration to those in a persistent vegetative state (2007). Even that clarification uses language of "ordinary and proportionate means of preserving life," which is consistent with Cronin's terminology.

Marking Archbishop Cronin's anniversaries in 2008—the fiftieth anniversary of the original printing of his dissertation, the fiftieth anniversary of the awarding of his doctoral degree in sacred theology, and the fortieth anniversary of his ordination as a bishop—The National Catholic Bioethics Center is republishing *Ordinary and Extraordinary Means of Conserving Life* as a testament to the dedication of the Church to the scholarly pursuit of truth. As Pope John Paul II stated in *Fides et ratio* (1998), "Revelation ... introduces into our history a universal and ultimate truth which stirs the human mind to ceaseless effort; indeed, it impels reason continually to extend the range of its knowledge until it senses that it has done all in its power, leaving no stone unturned" (n. 15). The NCBC hopes that this fiftieth anniversary edition of *Ordinary and Extraordinary Means* will continue to assist others in the ceaseless pursuit of universal and ultimate moral truth.

Editor's Preface

When he was a young graduate student, Archbishop Daniel A. Cronin had the opportunity to carry out research for his doctoral dissertation at the Vatican Library, were he examined the distinction between ordinary and extraordinary means. Perhaps the remarkable documents he had in his hands will be made more widely available in the future, but until they are they will be inaccessible to most of us. Cronin had a unique opportunity to study the great theologians of the late Middle Ages and early modern periods and put his scholarly skills to excellent use.

One of the many striking aspects of Cronin's survey is the consistency and agreement among past theologians. These men were not seeking to "push the envelope," as do many of our contemporary bioethicists, who are perhaps more interested in gaining tenure or public recognition than in providing genuine assistance to those facing difficult medical decisions. The bioethicists of that time, if the contemporary term may be applied, saw themselves as part of an ongoing philosophical tradition that sought to give good counsel on questions concerning the use of medical techniques that were, in most cases, far more primitive than those we are fortunate to have today. The medieval and early modern theologians took a commonsense approach to these decisions.

Cronin's dissertation is a superb historical survey, but given how rapidly medicine is evolving, it is also an interesting historical document itself. The work appeared in the 1950s, and it is striking to see how much things have changed in little more than a half century. Some of these changes are social, others economic. For example, many physicians of that time thought that there was a duty to do whatever was possible to preserve the life of the patient. That attitude, along with a highly pronounced paternalism, was already being questioned by the middle of the twentieth century, as Cronin's book makes clear. Having reviewed historical teaching on the difference between ordinary and extraordinary means, Cronin was well positioned to counsel physicians against this "life at all costs" attitude. The physician has no moral obligation, he writes, to use all available means to extend life, but only the obligation to use those measures that constitute ordinary means of treatment.

Cronin also recognizes the growing relevance of the psychological factor (*vehemens horror*) in making medical decisions. Amputation, which served as the most common example of an extraordinary means of treatment throughout much of the medieval and early modern periods, was no longer deemed extraordinary by the mid-nineteenth century. With the discoveries of anesthesia and antisepsis, the procedure was not nearly as painful or as dangerous as it had been previously. Nonetheless, Cronin holds that amputation may very well remain an extraordinary measure if the patient deems it too distressing psychologically. This could easily be the case, he suggests, if both legs were to be removed. Even with the advent of prostheses, radical disfigurement is naturally horrifying.

We forget how dramatically anesthesia redrew the medical landscape. With the appearance of effective painkillers, many procedures that previously had been deemed extraordinary became ordinary means of treatment. Anesthesiology not only reduced suffering, but caused dangerous surgical procedures to become virtually routine practices. The change in medical thinking occurred swiftly, though there was considerable initial resistance to moving many of these invasive surgeries from the category of the extraordinary to the ordinary. Here physicians led the way, rather than theologians.

The debate over the provision of nutrition and hydration to patients was also very much under discussion when Cronin's book was first published. There was vigorous disagreement over whether the provision of food and water to patients in seriously compromised cerebral conditions was obligatory, and Cronin cites the competing opinions. Cronin takes an open-ended view of the matter, which must now be tempered by recent statements from the Congregation for the Doctrine of the Faith. In assessing his judgment on this difficult question, we should bear in mind that the methods for providing food and water for patients in these conditions has much improved, thus changing the relevant circumstances.

A rather astonishing aspect of Cronin's book is its reports on the costs of medical care during the 1950s. These costs seem laughably low. For example, the cost of care for a patient with acute appendicitis, including anesthesia, medication, and an eight-day hospital stay, was only $133. That is unimaginable today. Elsewhere, Cronin observes that the moral theologians of his time generally agreed that a cost of $2,000 for a medical procedure was far too high to be obligatory. Such a figure would hardly cause one to bat an eye today. Once again, we see that the line between ordinary and extraordinary means changes continually.

The heart of the book, and its most rewarding feature, is its broad sweep of historical opinion. Under the heading "the malice of suicide," Cronin begins his research with a discussion of the general duty to conserve one's life, for the duty to conserve life follows from the obligation not to kill ourselves. Thomas Aquinas serves as the starting point for this discussion. God, Thomas says, is master over life and death (*Summa theologiae* II–II, q. 64, a. 5). We are not to decide the moment when we pass from this world to the next. To preserve ourselves in existence is a fundamental and inviolable law of our human nature.

Cronin discusses cases that would appear to be exceptions to this rule, but which are in fact actions justifiable under the principle of double effect. These are often cast before us as if they were serious objections to the duty to preserve our lives, but Cronin shows, for example, that the willingness of the soldier to die in battle for others does not contradict this principle. The same holds true for one who chooses to care for those infected with a contagious disease despite great danger to his or her own life.

Arguably, Francisco de Vitoria, OP, was the first to lay out the distinction between ordinary and extraordinary means, though he did not use these terms himself. He focused instead on the duty of using commonly available drugs and foods to preserve one's health. Later thinkers developed these themes under the headings that we have come to recognize today; their names constitute a who's who of great theological minds: Domingo de Soto, OP, Gregory Sayrus, OSB, Domingo Bañez, OP, Tomás Sánchez, SJ, Francisco Suarez, SJ, Juan de Lugo, SJ, Benoît Merkelbach, OP, Marcelino Zalba, SJ, and Gerald Kelly, SJ, to mention only the most prominent.

To illustrate an excessive burden, Cardinal de Lugo provides us with the hypothetical case of the man condemned to death by fire. If he were to find himself in possession of a sufficient amount of water to put out part of the fire, but not all of it, he would not be obliged to use the water at all.

Use would only prolong an inevitable death. Cronin's book also discusses the problem of excessive expense. Although we may at times today shy away from the idea that monetary considerations should play a role in health care decisions, the problem of cost has been a prominent feature of this discussion throughout history.

The most valuable feature of Cronin's work is its description of the various categories used by the theologians to differentiate ordinary and extraordinary means. The common headings for ordinary means handed down to us are "what provides hope of benefit," "means in common use," "means in keeping with one's status in life," and "means that are not too difficult." The common headings for extraordinary means are "what is impossible," "what requires great effort or excessive hardship," "what causes excruciating or excessive pain," "what causes feelings of intense fear or repugnance," and "means that involve extraordinary expense."

Cronin notes that it is not possible to identify an absolute standard for either ordinary or extraordinary means. The determination is specific to context. We cannot say, for example, what will be ordinary or extraordinary for human nature as such. There is no absolute moral norm. We can arrive at only a general standard that would apply to a majority of human beings, but such a standard admits of exceptions by its very nature. The distinction between ordinary and extraordinary means of treatment is best characterized, therefore, as a relative standard that must be adjusted to the particulars of a given patient, time, and situation.

The final chapter of Cronin's dissertation concerns the physician's duties to patients. There is a moral obligation to care for the sick that flows from the virtues of charity and justice. The content of this duty consists primarily of the obligation to employ the ordinary means of conserving life, but it may also extend to an obligation to use extraordinary means if this is the wish of the patient or the family; however,

Cronin warns the physician not to employ extraordinary means unless specifically asked to do so. This advice went against an all-too-common attitude of the time when the dissertation was first published. Most physicians today would not think that they have an obligation, regardless of the prospects for success, to use all available means of preserving life.

In the first (1989) edition of this work by The National Catholic Bioethics Center (then called the Pope John XXIII Medical-Moral Research and Education Center), Cronin's dissertation was bound together with two other important monographs on related topics: "Feeding the Hopeless and the Helpless," by Rev. Msgr. Orville N. Griese, STD, JCD, and "The Moral Option Not to Conserve Life under Certain Conditions," by Rev. Albert Moraczewski, OP, PhD. Despite the continued relevance of these works, we have decided that Archbishop Cronin's contribution merits its own self-standing publication.

To this day, we continue to receive requests for copies of Cronin's treatise. We are convinced that this reprinting will once again find an eager audience. For those familiar with the previous edition, we have made several improvements. The table of contents has been simplified, spelling and punctuation have been updated, and dates for the lives of the major theologians have been provided. The excellent table that Cronin provided in the first edition has been recast in a clearer format. The original appendices are included here, but in proper chronological order.

I would like to say a word of personal thanks to Dr. Marie Hilliard for writing the foreword to this new edition. Dr. Hilliard is a lifelong friend of Archbishop Cronin. The two forged a strong professional relationship during the time that Dr. Hilliard worked diligently with him on matters of public policy for the Archdiocese of Hartford.

Editor's Preface

For those interested in the historical development of the distinction between ordinary and extraordinary means, it would be hard to find a more important or comprehensive work. The depth of the research alone is invaluable, but when combined with Cronin's own insights into the application of this vital distinction to particular issues and cases, one has in hand a truly remarkable work.

EDWARD J. FURTON
Director of Publications
The National Catholic Bioethics Center

Preface to the New Edition

Fifty years after the publication of my dissertation, *The Moral Law in Regard to the Ordinary and Extraordinary Means of Conserving Life*, as part of a requirement for the doctoral degree in sacred theology at the Gregorian University in Rome, I have the happy privilege of writing these words as a foreword to the new edition of this work. In 1988, the Pope John XXIII Center—now The National Catholic Bioethics Center—incorporated the dissertation into a volume titled *Conserving Human Life*. Twenty years later, the NCBC is publishing the dissertation anew under the title *Ordinary and Extraordinary Means of Conserving Life*.

I remain surprised, as I stated at the time of the earlier publication, that my dissertation should have become such a valuable and useful resource for scholars doing important research on the many bioethical dilemmas encountered in contemporary health care delivery. If this new edition can aid in the furtherance of a proper appreciation of the value of human life and the obligation of each human being to preserve his or her life with the appropriate means, then all the long and tedious research that went into the original dissertation was worthwhile.

Preface to the New Edition

I renew my expression of gratitude to those whom I originally thanked, including the late Monsignor Orville Griese, whose insistent encouragement was the main reason for my agreeing to the 1988 publication of the dissertation, and to the National Catholic Bioethics Center. In particular, it must be noted that none of this would have occurred if it were not for the generosity of the Most Reverend Richard J. Cushing, then Archbishop of Boston, who assigned me to study for the doctoral degree in sacred theology. It is my hope and prayer that this new edition of *Ordinary and Extraordinary Means of Conserving Life* will continue to assist scholars in their pursuit of moral truth.

Most Reverend Daniel A. Cronin, STD
Archbishop Emeritus of the
Archdiocese of Hartford
December 20, 2008

Preface to the Dissertation

Father Cronin, then a priest of the Archdiocese of Boston, defended his dissertation in 1956, and it was published in 1958. This is his preface to that publication.

This dissertation is the study of the moral law in regard to the ordinary and extraordinary means of conserving life. The moral principles of the natural law which govern the actions of men are immutable. However, as years pass, these moral principles must be applied. But before these principles can be applied to the new conditions, it is very often necessary to investigate the meaning and implications of the principles. When the principles themselves are thus understood, an application of them to practical cases in new circumstances is not only easier but more exact.

This is particularly true in regard to the moral teaching on the ordinary and extraordinary means of conserving life. The advance of medical science presents in these days moral problems never before envisioned. Yet these modern problems can be solved with the correct application of basic and changeless moral principles if these principles are well understood. Very often medico-moral problems concern the licitness of a particular method of medical procedure. The moral solution in these cases concerns an action which may or may not be posited. However, the moral law in regard to the ordinary and extraordinary means of conserving life centers on a positive obligation. It concerns the definite duty incumbent on all men to care for their lives and health.

Modern medical science has advanced greatly. Today it provides many artificial methods of preservation and prolongation of life. Very often these methods are successful, often they are accompanied by serious danger and risk, often they are unsuccessful. Hence, an obvious question arises in regard to the moral obligation of using these means of conserving life. This moral question is especially pertinent when medical science is unable to cure a particular disease but is able to postpone the death caused by the disease.

The textbooks and manuals of moral theology distinguish the ordinary means of conserving life from the extraordinary means of conserving life. The ordinary means are morally obligatory means, and the extraordinary means are usually not morally obligatory. The discussions on this question found in the manuals of moral theology, however, are quite brief. In general, they merely summarize the teaching found in the writings of the moralists of the sixteenth and seventeenth centuries, and very few authors have made any attempt to study this problem in the light of modern medical progress.

Before any licit application of the teachings of the moralists in this matter can be made to present-day problems, one must clearly understand what the moralists mean by the terms "ordinary means of conserving life" and "extraordinary means of conserving life." The early moralists did not define these terms, and they rarely, if ever, explained them. Frequently, however, they gave elements which constituted for them ordinary means and extraordinary means. Frequently too they gave examples of ordinary and extraordinary means.

Preface to the Dissertation

In the first chapter of this dissertation, the reader will find a study of the basic duty that binds all men to conserve their lives. This study is a necessary prerequisite to any discussion of the ordinary and extraordinary means of conserving life.

The second chapter contains an historical report of the opinion of the most noteworthy moral theologians in regard to the ordinary and extraordinary means of conserving life. Since many of these treatments cannot be found in the modern manuals of moral theology, they are given in chapter 2 as a basis for the discussion of these opinions, which follows in chapter 3.

The first part of chapter 3 contains an analysis of the opinions of the moralists in regard to the ordinary and extraordinary means of conserving life. With the aid of this analysis, an attempt is then made to determine the nature of the ordinary and extraordinary means of conserving life. In the second part of the third chapter, a discussion of the moral obligation of using the ordinary and extraordinary means of conserving life is found.

The fourth chapter contains practical considerations in regard to the teaching on the ordinary and extraordinary means of conserving life, particularly with reference to modern medical and surgical procedures, and the obligation of the doctor in regard to supplying the ordinary and extraordinary means when he is treating a patient.

This dissertation is not a medical study of the ordinary and extraordinary means of conserving life. Rather, it is a study of the moral law in regard to these means. Hence, this dissertation contains discussions on the history of the moral teaching in this matter, the nature of ordinary and extraordinary means, and the moral obligation of using these means. Since the manuals of moral theology present only a very limited treatment of this problem, and since the concept of the nature of the ordinary and extraordinary means of conserving life is not always clear, and finally, since the determination of the moral obligation of using these means can sometimes be involved, it is hoped that this dissertation will present some clarification in regard to this very interesting and timely moral problem. In this way, it is also hoped that the theological investigation of the moral teaching on the ordinary and extraordinary means of conserving life will have been furthered and any future applications to practical cases, occasioned by medical progress, will thus be facilitated.

The author wishes to express his sincere gratitude to His Excellency The Most Rev. Richard J. Cushing, DD, Archbishop of Boston, for the opportunity to undertake graduate studies in sacred theology. Thanks are also due to Thomas P. Linehan Jr., MD, of London, whose advice and suggestions have been of great assistance. The author is particularly indebted to the late Rev. Edwin F. Healey, SJ, professor of moral theology for many years at the Pontifical Gregorian University in Rome, for his generous and expert guidance in directing the writing of this dissertation.[1]

Daniel A. Cronin
1958

---

[1] The author holds in prayerful remembrance his mother and father, to whom the original dissertation was dedicated.

Ordinary and Extraordinary Means of Conserving Life

Chapter 1

The Duty to Conserve Life

Human life is at once a gift and a responsibility—a gift because man could never create himself; a responsibility because man must use this gift properly. God, Life itself, is the source of all other life, and to Him alone, therefore, belongs every power over it. Christians have ever appreciated this truth, and none perhaps better than the Apostle Paul: "None of us lives as his own master and none of us dies as his own master. While we live we are responsible to the Lord, and when we die we die as his servants. Both in life and in death we are the Lord's."[1]

Among the natural gifts with which the Most High God has favored man, there is none so excellent as that of life, because it is life that is the basis for all that man has or can hope to attain.

The human person exists as a composite: the immortal soul by which he is endowed with an intellect and free will (this makes him similar to God Himself), and the body through which his soul acts to satisfy man's natural needs and to acquire merit in the supernatural order.

---

[1] Rom. 14:7–8.

Human life then is a gift, the fuller meaning of which becomes more evident elsewhere in Catholic theology. For the moral theologian, however, the aspect of main concern is life as a responsibility. This dissertation will treat of one point under that aspect, namely, the extent to which man has the duty of conserving his corporeal life here in this world. In other words, presupposing the fact that on earth the body is a necessity in order that "the man" can act, this investigation will continue on then to determine just what responsibility man has to conserve his bodily life and health prior to that final hour which God alone knows and He alone will divulge.

THE MALICE OF SUICIDE

Interestingly enough, the reasons traditionally assigned to prove the duty of self-conservation are the very same ones by which the theologians have consistently exposed the basic malice of suicide. To explain, therefore, that suicide is evil is by that very fact a virtual demonstration of an equally true proposition: self-conservation is a duty.

It is quite apparent that there exists deeply embedded in the human fiber a strong drive which urges man on to self-conservation. Gradually, it also becomes clear that there is coupled together with this human urge a very definite duty to conserve one's life. Nonetheless, however forceful the natural drive may be, or however clear the duty of self-conservation may become, one seeks an explanation of the underlying reasons, and this can be involved.

Quite often it happens that before any process of reasoning takes place, one recognizes the truth of the conclusion. It is only when the intellect brings forth the arguments that the difficulty begins. This detail did not escape the eminent Cardinal Juan de Lugo, S.J. (1583–1660); it is precisely in his discussion of suicide that he mentions it.[2] For de Lugo, the intrinsic wickedness of suicide is immediately apparent; the basis of this truth, however, is not quite so obvious.

Scripture, the Fathers, and the Church

Properly speaking, suicide, as understood here, is the direct killing of a man, perpetrated by the man himself and on his own authority.[3] Suicide, thus understood, is always gravely illicit.

That God alone has the power of life and death, the Book of Deuteronomy clearly states: "Learn then that I, I alone, am God, and there is no god besides me. It is I who bring both death and life."[4] And again in Wisdom: "For you have dominion over life and death; you lead down to the gates of the nether world, and lead back."[5]

To God then, belongs the power of life, and man must never fancy that he may determine the hour of death—

---

[2] "Tota difficultas consistit in assignanda ratione huius veritatis: nam licet turpitudo haec statim appareat, non tamen facile est eius fundamentum invenire: unde, quod in aliis multis quaestionibus contingit, magis certa est conclusio, quam rationes, quae variae a diversis afferuntur ad eius probationem." J. de Lugo, *Disputationes scholasticae et morales* (Paris, 1868–1869), VI, *De iustitia a iure*, disp. X, sec. I, n. 2.

[3] Later in this discussion, the broader definition as given in E. F. Regatillo and M. Zalba, *Theologiae moralis summa* (Madrid: Biblioteca de Autores Cristianos, 1953; hereafter Regatillo-Zalba), II, p. 257, will prove more accurate. Zalba, the author of this second volume, defines suicide as "actio vel ommisio quae ad mortem propriam causandam natura sua ordinata."

[4] Deut. 32:39.

[5] Wisd. 16:13.

Thou shalt not kill.[6] By this fifth injunction of the Decalogue, God forbids not only homicide but also suicide. How cleverly St. Augustine caught the full import of the fifth commandment:

> It is not without significance, that in no passage of the holy canonical books can there be found either divine precept or permission to take away our own life whether for the sake of entering on the enjoyment of immortality or of shunning or ridding ourselves of anything whatever. Nay, the law, rightly interpreted even prohibits suicide where it says, Thou shalt not kill. This is proved specially by the omission of the words, "thy neighbor," which are inserted when false witness is forbidden ... how much greater reason have we to understand that a man may not kill himself, since in the commandment, "Thou shalt not kill," there is no limitation added nor any exception made in favour of anyone, at least of all in favour of him on whom the command is laid. ... The commandment is "Thou shalt not kill man"—therefore neither another nor yourself, for he who kills himself still kills nothing else than man.[7]

Such has been the tradition among ecclesiastical writers through the ages, as these excerpts testify:

> For if the one guilty of homicide is wicked because he destroys a man, the same crime is to be leveled on him who kills himself because he also kills a man. Indeed, we must consider this crime greater, the revenge for which lies with God alone. For, just as we did not come into this life of our own

---

[6]Exod. 20:13.

[7]Augustine, *De civitate Dei*, lib. 1, cap. 20, in *Patrologiae cursus completus, series latina* (Paris: Migne, 1844–1864; hereafter Migne, PL), 41.34–35. The translation of this passage is by Marcus Dods, from the Modern Library edition of *City of God* (New York: Random House, 1950).

free-will, so also we must leave this domicile of the body, which was given to us to watch over, by the command of the same person who placed us in this body to inhabit it until such time as He orders us to depart from it.[8]—LACTANTIUS (ca. 320)

It is not up to us to seize death but to accept it willingly when inflicted by others.[9]—ST. JEROME (d. 420)

Excepting those whom either a generally just law or the very source of justice, God, in a special way commands to be killed, anyone who would kill another man or himself is guilty of the crime of homicide.[10]— RABANUS MAURUS (d. 856)

Peter Abelard (1079–1142) also discusses the problem of suicide in chapter 155 of his *Theologica et philosophica*, giving many famous examples from ancient times.[11]

---

[8] "Nam si homicida nefarius est, quia hominis exstinctor est, eidem sceleri obstrictus est, qui se necat, quia hominem necat. Imo vero maius esse id facinus existimandum est, cuius ultio Deo soli subiacet. Nam sicut in hanc vitam non nostra sponte venimus, ita rursus ex hoc domicilio corpus induxit, tamdiu habituros, donec iubeat emitti." Lactantius, *Divinarum institutionum*, lib. III., cap. 18 (Migne, PL 6.407).

[9] "Non est nostrum, mortem arripere, sed illatam ab aliis libenter excipere." Jerome, *Commentaria in Jonam*, cap. 1, ver. 12 (Migne, PL 25.1129).

[10] "His ergo exceptis quos vel lex generaliter iusta vel ipse fons iustitiae Deus specialiter occidi iubet, quisquis hominem vel seipsum vel quemlibet occiderit, homicidii crimine innecitur. " Rabanus Maurus, *Commentaria in libros machabaeorum* (Migne, PL 109.1255).

[11] P. Abelard, *Theologica et philosophica* (Migne, PL 178.1603–1606). See also "Index de suicidio," Migne, PL 220.858–861, for a concise list of other references to the crime of suicide in the writings of the ecclesiastical authors.

The teaching of the Church has been no less constant. Even in the sixth century, the church legislated against suicide in the Council of Orleans.[12] It was decided at that time not to accept the offerings of a man who died by his own hand. In the catechism of the Council of Trent, one reads, "No man possesses such power over his life as to be at liberty to put himself to death. Hence we find that the commandment does not say: Thou shalt not kill another, but simply Thou shalt not kill."[13] More recently, Pope Leo XIII reiterated the Church's doctrine when writing to the Bishops of Germany and Austria in regard to dueling.[14] Add to this also the sanctions placed on the one who had attempted suicide ("sibi vitam adimere tentaverit") by the laws of the Church in the present *Codex iuris canonici*,[15] and it then becomes quite clear that the teaching of the Church holds suicide to be a grave sin.

St. Thomas and Subsequent Theologians

Catholic theologians have ever been mindful of the problem of suicide and in their writings have constantly

---

[12] J. Mansi, *Sacrorum conciliorum nova et amplissima collectio*, ed. nov. (Florence, 1759–1798), VIII, 837.

[13] "Neque vero seipsum interficere cuipiam fas est; cum vitae suae nemo ita potestatem habeat, ut suo arbitratu mortem sibi consciscere liceat, ideoque huius Legis verbis non ita preascriptum est, Ne alium occidas, sed simpliciter, Ne occidas." *Catechismus ex decreto SS Concilii Tridentini* (Padua, 1758), pars tertia, cap. VI, de quinto praecepto, n. 10.

[14] Leo XIII, *Pastoralis officii*, epistola ad episcopos Germ. et Austr., September 12, 1891, in H. Denzinger, *Enchiridion symbolorum*, ed. J. Umberg (Freiburg: Herder, 1942; hereafter Denzinger), n. 1939.

[15] *Code of Canon Law*, Latin–English edition (Washington, D.C.: Canon Law Society of America, 1983), cann. 1041.5 and 1044.3.

censured it as base and despicable, always and everywhere to be condemned. The arguments employed by the theologians have their foundation in Sacred Scripture, the writings of the Fathers and Doctors of the Church, the practice of the Church, and also in reason itself.

St. Thomas (1225–1274) had an extraordinary understanding of metaphysics and thus produced an equally extraordinary treatment of ethics.[16] Hence, his tract on suicide in question 64, article 5, of the Secunda Secundae of his *Summa theologica* has been the basis for the subsequent theological discussions on the subject down through the years.

After introducing this article, as is his wont, with five arguments in favor of the opposite opinion, St. Thomas proceeds to demonstrate by a threefold argument of the malice of suicide. First of all, suicide is against the natural inclination and charity with which everyone should love himself. In the second place, since every man is a part of the community and in that sense belongs to the community, he does an injury to the community when he destroys himself. Lastly, since God alone, according to Scripture, causes a man to live, and He alone should decide the hour of death, the one who deprives himself of life by suicide is actually usurping the judgment of a matter over which God actually never gave him jurisdiction.[17] St. Thomas, replying to the first objection, adds that suicide has a double aspect: in relation to the man himself,

---

[16] See G. Gustafson, *The Theory of Natural Appentency in the Philosophy of St. Thomas* (Washington, D.C.: Catholic University Press, 1944), p. 99.

[17] Thomas Aquinas, *Summa theologiae* (Turin: Marietti, 1950; hereafter *Summa theologiae*) II-II, q. 64, art. 5. For a very good commentary on this article, see *Somme théologique de Saint Thomas D'Aquin*, edition de la Revue des Jeunes (Paris: Desclée, 1934), II, *La justice*, pp. 146ss.

the guilty party has sinned against charity; in relation to God and the community, he has sinned against justice.[18]

Is man the master of himself? If so, it would seem that he might choose to live or die. Hence, any attempt on his part to appoint the hour of death would not only be licit, but sometimes, might even be laudable; e.g., he could select the time when his soul would be best prepared to meet God and thus insure his salvation. At least, one must admit that by suicide, if it were licit, it would be possible to avoid further sin.

Contained in the above reasoning is a fallacy which the Angelic Doctor exposes in his reply to the third objection:

> We must say that man is constituted master of himself by his free will. Of his own free will, therefore, man is allowed to dispose of things of his life. But the passage from this life to a happier life, does not lie within the power of man's free will but, rather, within the power of Almighty God.[19]

Theologians subsequent to St. Thomas were heavily influenced by his argumentation. Some, in fact, were content with either a direct quoting of his words or a mere rephrasing.[20] Others, however, began to consider the full import of the reasoning, and thus, have left in their works a heritage of further thought on the subject. For example, the notion of justice existing between God and man was the point that

---

[18] *Summa theologiae* II-II, q. 64, art. 5, ad 1.

[19] "Ad tertium dicendum quod homo constituitur dominus sui ipsius per liberum arbitrium. Et ideo licite potest homo de seipso disponere quantum ad ea quae pertinent ad hanc vitam, quae hominis libero arbitrio regitur. Sed transitus de hac vita ad aliam feliciorem non subiacet libero arbitrio hominis, sed potestati divinae." Ibid., ad 3.

[20] See D. Soto, *De justitia et jure* (Lyon, 1582), lib. V, q. I, art. V.

Luis de Molina, S.J. (1535–1600) found troublesome. For him, our relationship with God is not one of justice; at least it does not fulfill the complete notion of justice because we are never in the position of being able to render to God the equivalent of what He gives us. However, Molina feels that even though there is something of higher value than justice which binds us to God, nevertheless, we can speak of justice in the less strict sense,[21] and thus condemns suicide as a sin against justice with respect to God.[22] This is true because man does not possess dominion over his own life; the Author of nature has reserved this dominion to Himself.[23]

When one is said to have dominion over anything, the implication is that he has supreme authority over it.[24] Hence, when theologians repeat again and again that the dominion over life belongs to God, they mean that He alone has the supreme and ultimate power over it.[25]

On this notion of dominion, theologians have built their argument from reason. De Lugo develops it nicely. The Cardinal cites the statement of St. Thomas in the *Summa theologica* II-II, q. 64, art. 5, that man is not the master of his life. Then de Lugo proceeds to praise Molina for a very fine exposition of the consequence of this statement. Since man is not the master of his life, he cannot dispose of it at will; much less can he destroy it, because to destroy something implies an act which is proper only to the one having supreme mastery

---

[21] See *Summa theologiae* II-II, q. 58, a. 2.

[22] See L. Molina, *De iustitia et iure* (Cologne, 1614), tom. IV, tract. III, disp. 1, n. 1.

[23] Ibid., disp. 9, n. 2. Also *Summa theologiae* II-II, q. 59, art. 3, ad 2.

[24] See *Webster's Collegiate Dictionary*, s.v. "dominion" (Springfield, MA: Merriam Co., 1942), p. 299.

[25] See Deut. 32:39.

over it. This is all well and good, but for de Lugo, the problem is not explaining the consequence but rather proving the fact that man is not master of his own life. Very cleverly, de Lugo goes to the heart of the argumentation. For him, therefore, once it is proved that man does not possess supreme authority over his life, then everything else fits into place—but first, prove the point:

> Now we prove that man is not the master of his life this way: Although man can receive dominion over things which are extrinsic to himself or which are distinct from him, he cannot, however, receive dominion over himself, because from the very concept and definition, it is clear that a master is something relative, for example, a father or a teacher; and just as no one can be father or teacher of himself, so neither can he be master of himself, for to be master always denotes superiority with regard to the one over whom he is the master. Hence, God Himself cannot be master of Himself, even though He possesses Himself most perfectly. Therefore man cannot be master of himself; however, he can be master of his operations, and therefore, he can sell himself and thus, improperly speaking, we might say he gives mastery of himself to another but, he really does not give over mastery of himself basically or radically, but only mastery over certain of his operations, ... therefore a man can dispose only of his own operations of which he is the master, not of himself (or to say the same thing), not of his own life over which he is not master, nor can he be.[26]

---

[26] "Porro hominem non esse dominum suae vitae, probari potest, quia licet homo potuerit accipere dominium aliarum rerum, quae sunt extra ipsum, vel quae ab ipso distinguuntur; non tamen potuit accipere dominium sui ipsius, quia ut ex ipso conceptu et definitione constat, dominus est aliquid relativum, sicut pater, et

A study of these words of de Lugo's reveals that fundamentally, he bases his reasoning on the notion of relativity contained in the concept of dominion, and ultimately on the relation which man, the creature, has to God, his Creator. For de Lugo, to have dominion necessarily implies something extrinsic to the one having dominion. Over and above that, dominion implies superiority, so that not even God has dominion over Himself, properly speaking. Since it is obvious that no man can be extrinsic or superior to himself, it follows that neither can he be basically master or lord of himself in regard to his life.

While it is true that man possesses a mastery over the actions of his life, which after all proceed from his own free will, he does not possess any like mastery over his life radically. Therefore, lacking the mastery, he must not act the part of a master and perform an act proper to the master alone—destruction. Hence, because of the lack of dominion in the strict sense, direct suicide is gravely illicit.[27]

---

magister; quare sicut nemo potest esse pater vel magister sui ipsius, ita nec potest esse sui ipsius dominus: nam dominus semper dicit superiotitatem respectu illius cuius est dominus, ita nec potest esse sui ipsius, ita nec potest esse sui ipsius dominus. Unde nec Deus ipse potest esse dominus sui ipsius, quamvis possideat perfectissime seipsum. Non potuit ergo homo fieri dominus sui ipsius, potest quidem esse dominus suarum operationum, et ideo potest vendere seipsum, et tunc dicitur improprie dare aleri dominium sui ipsius; sed revera non dat proprie dominium sui simpliciter sed solum in ordine ad aliquas suas operationes ... solum ergo potest homo disponere de suis operationibus, quarum dominus est, non de seipso, vel, quod idem est, de vita sua, cuius dominus non est, nec esse potest." De Lugo, *De iustitia a iure*, disp. X, sec. I, n. 9.

[27] See ibid., n. 10ff., where de Lugo refutes the objections made to his doctrine.

Who, then, has the supreme dominion? The implication is rather simple for de Lugo. God is the only one who is both extrinsic and superior to man—it is from God that man came—and, therefore, He alone has supreme dominion. This becomes clear from de Lugo's reply to the first objection where he reasons that it would be licit for a man to kill himself in virtue of a precept or permission from God, because God, after all, possesses the most perfect dominion over life and man would act then as his instrument.[28]

The theologians appreciated the value of this basic notion of dominion. It was quite logical then for them to take the next step and apply the distinction existing at the time in juridic terminology between dominion over the "substance" of a thing and dominion over its "usefulness." The first is known as a direct or radical dominion; the second as an indirect dominion or dominion of use.[29] With these terms, then, the theologians explained the difference between God's status and man's status in regard to a man's human life. To God belongs the basic or radical dominion, and He allows man an indirect dominion or possession of its usefulness. Regarding his human life, man has only the right to its proper use, because God alone possesses the basic lordship over its substance.

It is in this manner that for centuries theologians have refuted the arguments in favor of suicide and proved its malice. The reasoning can be put in the form of traditional scholastic argumentation as follows:

> Man in killing himself usurps the direct dominion over his life which belongs to God alone. To usurp this dominion is a grave violation of a divine right.

---

[28] Ibid., n. 10.

[29] See F. Hürth and P. Abellán, *De praeceptis* (Rome: Pontificia Universitas Gregoriana, 1948), p. 20, for a brief but precise explanation of these juridic terms.

Therefore, man in killing himself violates in a serious way a divine right.

The proof then of the major is: the one having dominion over anything is the one for whom the usefulness of such a thing is primarily intended, so that he can dispose of it for his own benefit without fear of violating another man's prior rights. Man, however, has not been created primarily for his own convenience or utility, but rather for the glory and worship of God. Thus, he cannot dispose of himself without consideration of God's rights. Therefore, he is not his own master in regard to the basic rights over his life. The minor in the argumentation is clear enough, and discussion concerns only the major.

Such is the argumentation that appears generally in the writing of the Catholic theologians and moral philosophers.[30] True, changes here and there in the presentation of the argument occur. The variation depends on the author. No change, however, is so singular as to warrant special mention here. These writers in their expression of the argument based

---

[30] Alphonsus, *Theologica moralis* (Rome: Typographica Vaticana, 1948), lib. III, tract. 4, cap. 1, dub. 1, n. 366; A. Lehmkuhl, *Theologia moralis*, 10th ed. (Freiburg: Herder, 1902), I, pp. 346–347; H. Noldin and A. Schmitt, *Summa theologiae moralis*, 27th ed. (Innsbruck: Rauch, 1940–41; hereafter Noldin-Schmitt), II, p. 309; J. Aertnys and C. Damen, *Theologiae moralis*, 16th ed. (Turin: Marietti, 1950; hereafter Aertnys-Damen), I, p. 458; L. Fanfani, *Manuale theorico-practicum theologiae moralis* (Rome: Liberaria Ferrari, 1950), II, p. 323; Regatillo-Zalba, *Theologiae moralis summa*, II, p. 258; V. Cathrein, *Philosophia moralis*, 20th ed. (Freiburg: Herder, 1955), p. 245; J. B. Schuster, *Philosophia moralis* (Freiburg: Herder, 1950); J. Costa-Rossetti, *Philosophia moralis* (Innsbruck: Rauch, 1886), pp. 265ss; T. Meyer, *Institutiones iuris naturalis* (Freiburg: Herder, 1900), II, p. 41; and Iesus Iturrioz et al., *Philosophiae scholasticae summa* (Madrid: Biblioteca de Autores Cristianos, 1952), III, p. 553.

on the divine dominion over human life obviously suppose the existence of God, creation, and the end of man which is to be attained in the next life as facts proved elsewhere.[31] They then proceed to set forth their argument. This procedure is, of course, legitimate enough. As a matter of fact, the suppositions are quite necessary if one is to capture the validity of the reasoning process.[32]

One frequently finds the argument from charity conjoined with the argument based on the exclusive dominion of God over human life. Man is bound to exercise the virtue of charity in regard to himself as he is in regard to others, and this virtue he violates seriously by suicide.[33] However the argument based on the virtue of charity does not seem to find unconditioned favor, because of what theologians feel is a lack of universality. For example, one might argue that a situation could arise in which a man would actually show more love for himself if he would kill himself, rather than live in the necessary proximate danger of sinning seriously. Thus the authors feel that the prohibition against suicide must be proved from some other source besides the virtue of charity alone.[34] Once suicide is proved illicit by another

---

[31] See Schuster, *Philosophia moralis*, p. 91.

[32] There are some who feel that there is apparent in the argument based on the dominion of God an unwarranted influence of "juridism." See L. Bender, "Organorum humanorum transplantatio," *Angelicum* 31 (April–June 1954), pp. 148–149. Of interest also is the contention of some that all the arguments against suicide are founded on—in fact ultimately resolve themselves into the argument based on—man's lack of perfect dominion over himself.

[33] See Matt. 22:39; also F. Hürth and P. Abellán, *De principiis* (Rome: Pontificia Universitas Gregoriana, 1948), p. 276.

[34] See Schuster, *Philosophia moralis*, p. 91.

argument—for example, the singular right which God has over human life—then, of course, it is true to say that man also sins against the love which he owes himself.[35]

An interesting treatment of this problem occurs in the writings of Arthur Vermeersch, S.J. (1858–1936). His approach is slightly different. Vermeersch states the arguments based on the dominion of God and the charity due one's self. He then proceeds to show that suicide also offends against the virtue of piety toward one's self.[36] Vermeersch explains this by pointing out that when a man commits suicide, he removes the fundamental condition of all worship—his life. By so doing, he fails to acknowledge his essential dependence on God, the Creator, and thus refuses to recognize his obligation to revere in himself the image of God from Whom he has come and to Whom, alone, belongs the dominion over his life.[37]

By way of summary then, we may say the Catholic position in regard to suicide is that a man always sins seriously when he attempts to take his life on his own authority. This is so because suicide is a grave infraction of the natural law, the divine positive law, and the ecclesiastical law. The natural law is violated because man has only the right of using his life and never possesses a radical dominion over the substance of it. Hence, by suicide, he usurps a divine right. Suicide is prohibited also by the divine law in view of the

---

[35] See *Summa theologiae* II-II, q. 64, art. 5.

[36] A. Vermeersch, *Theologiae moralis principia-responsa-consilia*, 3rd ed. (Rome: Pontificia Universitas Gregoriana, 1945), II, n. 296.

[37] See A. Vermeersch, *Quaestiones de virtutibus religonis et pietatis* (Bruges: Bayaert, 1912), p. 205 note 183, and p. 215 note 190 for an added treatment of this argument.

fifth commandment,[38] the duty of loving one's self,[39] and the open declaration in Scripture of God's dominion over life.[40] Finally, the ecclesiastical law forbids suicide, and thus the perpetrator offends against Church law. Add to this the constant teachings of the ecclesiastical writers, theologians, and moralists, and one understands plainly and appreciates fully the import of the teaching of the Church in this matter. Scripture,[41] Tradition, and the teaching Church all show the malice of suicide.

THE GENERAL RULE AND EXCEPTIONS

Since man does not have perfect dominion over his life, but only a right to its use, which he receives from God, it follows that he is bound to take proper care of it. Since he does not own his life, he must conserve it until such time as is indicated by the rightful owner.

Man does have dominion over his actions and even a certain dominion over his life and members, but only such as allows him certain limited rights: "Furthermore private men

---

[38] Exod. 20:13.

[39] Matt. 22:39.

[40] Deut. 32:39 and Wisd. 16:13.

[41] History reveals instances in which saints and martyrs threw themselves into fire or undertook other fatal tortures. Because of this, an objection often arises against the Church's condemnation of suicide. Also, in the Old Testament, Samson killed himself (Judg. 16:30), and yet St. Paul numbered him among the saints (Heb. 11:32). The interpretation of these events can be found in de Lugo, *De iustitia a iure*, disp. X, sec. I, n. 15, and Regatillo-Zalba, *Theologiae moralis summa*, II, p. 259. See also Augustine, *De civitate Dei*, cap. 21, and Aquinas, *Summa theologiae* II-II, q. 64, art. 5, ad 4. Briefly, we may say that these authors interpret the actions of the saints and martyrs and usually explain them as having occurred because of an erroneous conscience or a divine inspiration.

have no dominion over the members of their body other than that which pertains to their natural ends."[42] Lacking therefore the perfect dominion, he not only must not destroy his life, but he must conserve it in a positive manner. He is not the lord of his life but only its custodian, and thus, he has the obligation and responsibility of caring for what has been entrusted to his charge. As the administrator of his life, he has the duty to take the steps necessary for its conservation. To him has been given life, not to be lost but to be conserved.

If however, man fails in this regard; if man decides to disregard his responsibility of administration and custody; if man does not conserve his life, he then violates the same law which forbids him to kill himself: "The same precept which prohibits suicide also prescribes by that very fact, the conservation of one's life, since not to conserve one's life and to commit suicide are virtually the same."[43] Hence, there is no difficulty in recognizing the duty of conserving one's life as a rather obvious consequence of the doctrine that suicide is illicit. Also, from the realization that man is merely the custodian of his life, the inference is clear—namely, he must conserve it and care for it.

Catholic Teaching

In the Decalogue, no one can find this specific command: Thou shalt conserve thy life. Yet Sacred Scripture certainly extols the value of human life. God is the ultimate

---

[42] "Ceterum, quod ipsi privati homines in sui corporis membra dominatum alium non habeant, quam quid ad eorum naturales fines pertineat." Pius XI, *Casti connubii*, December 31, 1930, Denzinger 2246.

[43] "Idem praeceptum, quod prohibet sui occisionem, eo ipso praecipit etiam propriae vitae conservationem, cum virtualiter idem sit vitam non conservare et vitam sibi adimere." Noldin-Schmitt, *Summa theologiae moralis*, II, p. 307.

end of man and of his actions, so that in all his actions, he should direct himself to glorifying God and one day possessing Him.[44] Man accomplishes this end by the exercise of his powers and faculties. God has given certain natural gifts to man and, if he uses these properly, he will merit eternal salvation, thus giving glory to God and attaining the lasting possession of God.

Among these gifts of God, there is none more precious than life itself, for without life, there is no power or faculty or action. The first requirement, therefore, for man in order that he may merit heaven is life here on earth. Then, as a true steward, he supervises these gifts of his Master until the Master demands an accounting.[45] His time of existence here on earth becomes for him a period of probation. The entire New Testament portrays life as the time in which man must use the God-given talents[46] with which he can save his soul. Life is a period of sowing good seed in preparation for the harvest.[47] It is during life that man has the opportunity of working in the vineyard of the Lord.[48] Thus he is able to store up treasures in heaven.[49]

If, therefore, the relation between man's life on earth and future happiness in heaven is so intimate, an appreciation of the value of his life immediately arises. Man then should guard it, protect it, care for it, and conserve it as he would any precious thing. Certainly, he should not injure it; much less should he destroy it. However, since man in this present economy cannot hold himself indifferent to his

---

[44]Regatillo-Zalba, *Theologiae moralis summa*, I, pp. 36–44.
[45]Luke 16:2.
[46]Matt. 25:14–30.
[47]Matt. 13:24–30.
[48]Matt. 20:1.
[49]Matt. 6:20.

supernatural end which is obligatory,[50] and since this end is attained by the correct use of his powers and faculties here on earth, one can argue that, therefore, the use of these powers and faculties and the life which is their foundation is also obligatory, because he who is bound to an end is bound also to the means. Then, since the use of the means, which in this case have not been freely elected by man but assigned by God,[51] is obligatory, the conservation of them is also obligatory. This is true because the obligation to use a thing does not bind unless the thing exists. In this particular case, however, the thing concerned—his life and faculties—has been placed at man's disposal by a higher power precisely for that purpose, namely, use. Furthermore, it can be gathered from Sacred Scripture, as we saw above, that the time for meriting is not a period determined by the servant but rather by the Master. Thus, the use of necessary means of meriting and their conservation is obligatory not merely for a stated time, but until such time as God demands a settling of man's eternal account. Hence, it is true to say that the responsibility which man has to conserve his life is evident also in Scripture.

From another point of view, Pope Leo XIII, in his encyclical *Rerum novarum*, expresses the necessity of conserving one's life. Writing about the nature of human work, the Pope remarks that work is not only something personal but also something quite necessary, because it is the way in which man can care for his human life. To take care of one's life, the Pontiff emphasizes, is a demand of the very nature of things with which it is necessary to comply.[52] The Holy Father says, "Indeed, to remain in life is a duty common to

---

[50] See Regatillo-Zalba, *Theologiae moralis summa*, I, pp. 45ss.

[51] See Meyer, *Institutiones iuris naturalis*, II, p. 48.

[52] Leo XIII, *Rerum novarum*, Denzinger 1938c.

all—the non-fulfillment of which is a crime. Hence, the right of acquiring the goods by which life is sustained necessarily arises."[53] The teaching of Leo XIII, therefore, declares openly that the right to work exists precisely because man has the duty to conserve his life, which he accomplishes by means which his daily work provides.

In this matter, the doctrine of the Church and her theologians has been consistent and constant through the ages. This is not surprising because, first of all, the Church has always condemned suicide, as has been shown, and thus the logical concomitant, self-conservation, has been rather obvious. Secondly, because of the value of human life as a precious gift of God, and of its necessity for performing meritorious acts, the theologians have, as we shall see, constantly emphasized the responsibility of using the means of self-conservation. An understanding of creation, the value of man's body and soul, and his final end leaves room for no other doctrine in this regard.

Commonly, theologians are accustomed to use also the argument based on the virtue of charity.[54] Man is bound to love himself. Therefore, a fortiori, he must exercise charity in regard to his life, and thus he is bound to care for his life and conserve it as the means which serve for obtaining eternal salvation.[55] Most theologians, however, add this argument to the others by which they have already proved the necessity of self-conservation.[56]

---

[53] "Reapse manere in vita, commune singulis officium est, cui scelus est deesse. Hinc ius reperiendarum rerum, quibus vita sustentatur, necessario nascitur." Ibid.

[54] See *Summa theologiae* II-II, q. 25, art. 4–5.

[55] See Fanfani, *Manuale theorico-practicum theologiae moralis*, II, p. 126.

[56] The theologians are somewhat reserved about this argument. They feel it is valid as far as it goes but that it is not sufficiently

St. Thomas employed the argument from charity when emphasizing the import of the natural attachment that all men have to life: "It is by nature that everything loves itself so that everything conserves itself in being and resists, as far as it can, any corrupting influences. Therefore, he who kills himself, acts against a natural inclination and against the charity by which a man should love himself." [57] This excerpt from the *Summa theologica* serves well as an introduction to the argument based on man's natural desire to live. St. Thomas recognized the instincts that man finds within himself. In his writings, therefore, he was quick to reveal their fuller meaning and implications. Certainly, the first instinct of man is the attachment to life and the desire to live. In fact, it is the first instinct of all living being. Quite properly, someone has defined life as the internal power of development and of resistance to destruction. [58] Within himself, man senses a vigorous drive which urges him on to protect and perfect himself under all conditions and to oppose all powers bent on his destruction. Deep within himself, he senses a passionate urge to live. Even in times

---

universal to prove by itself the necessity of self-conservation. This point has been mentioned already in the discussion on suicide, but it is worthwhile here to call attention to the treatment in Cathrein, *Philosophia moralis*, p. 247, n. 347.

[57] "Naturaliter quaelibet res seipsam amat: et ad hoc pertinet quod quaelibet res naturaliter conservat se in esse et corrumpentibus resistit quamtum potest. Et ideo quod aliquis seipsum occidat est contra inclinationem naturalem, et contra caritatem, qua quilibet debet seipsum diligere." *Summa theologiae* II-II, q. 64, art. 5, in corp.

[58] "Pouvoir interne de développement et de résistance à la destruction." J. Leclercq, *Leçons de droit naturel* (Namur: Wesmael-Charlier, 1937), IV, *Les droits et devoirs individuels*, première partie, p. 182.

of adversity, his basic concern is the protection of his well-being, and the fear of his own destruction initiates violent reactions throughout his whole human structure. His is an ardent love of life and a forceful instinct to live—and this he shares with every member of the human race.

There is no doubt that this basic instinct within man manifests the law of nature for him. Such a design of nature he must not only approve but effectively obey. Hence, he has the obligation to comply with nature and conserve his life in a positive manner. Not to do so constitutes a crime against nature, since he is acting against a natural inclination placed in him by the Author of nature itself.[59] One author phrases it this way: It is impossible that any appetite set up in us by nature should be directed to any other thing than the fuller being of the individual. It is impossible that it should aim at nothingness or at destruction.[60] A simple glance at human life as it exists today in the world, and as it has existed since the beginning, reveals that what is said of the theory of this human desire to live and better one's self has also worked out in practice. Man and woman unite to initiate the family by which they actually perfect their own personalities in addition to accomplishing other ends. The families have formed society, and all society is directed not only to the perpetuation and conservation of the human race, but also to its betterment and development by enabling man to accomplish in society what he could not do alone. Certainly, society is not bent on the destruction of the human race. Society represents the inner feelings of each individual of which it is comprised, and thus represents the

---

[59] See R. P. Sertillanges, *La philosophie morale de Saint Thomas d'Aquin* (Paris: Aubier-Montaigne, 1946), p. 182.

[60] M. Cronin, *The Science of Ethics* (Dublin: Gill & Son, 1917), II, p. 53.

individual's desire for life, development, and perfection. If at times society fails in this regard, the reason does not lie in any basic drive or urge to self-destruction, but rather in ignorance, blindness, bad will, and the many other effects of sin. This is evident even in war itself. Although one segment of society does not hesitate to destroy another, yet each individual member of society fears self-destruction and aims at his own protection and conservation.

This theme runs through the works of St. Thomas, as these few examples, besides the one already quoted, demonstrate:

> It is natural for each individual to love his own life and things pertaining thereto, but in due measure: that they are loved not as if the end of life were rooted in them, but that they must be used in view of the ultimate end of life. Hence failure to love these things in due measure is contrary to the natural inclination, and consequently, a sin.[61]

> Love of self-preservation because of which the dangers of death are avoided, is much more connatural than any pleasures whatever of food or sex which are intended for the preservation of life. Hence, it is more difficult to conquer the fear of dangers of death, than the desire of pleasure in the matter of food and sex.[62]

---

[61] "Inditum autum est unicuique naturaliter ut propriam vitam amet, et ea quae ad ipsam ordinantur; tamen debito modo: ut scilicet amantur huiusmodi non quasi finis constituatur in eis, sed secundum quod eis utendum est propter ultimum finem. Unde quod aliquis deficiat a debito modo amoris ipsorum, est contra naturalem inclinationem: et per consequens est peccatum." *Summa theologiae* II-II, q. 126, art. 1.

[62] "Amor conservationis vitae, propter quam vitantur pericula mortis, est multo magis connaturalis quam quaecumque delectationes ciborum vel venereorum, quae ad conservationem

Particular nature is conservative of each individual as much as it can, hence it is beyond intention that it be deficient in conserving.[63]

And according to this all corruption and defect is against nature because a power of this type intends its existence and the conservation of that of which it is.[64]

Finally,

An act of this type, since one's intention is to conserve one's life, is not illicit because it is natural to everything to conserve itself in being in as much as it can.[65]

These citations from the writings of St. Thomas emphasize not only the strength of his arguments in the particular matter he is treating but also, the fact that all men sense within themselves a drive urging them on to the conservation of their own lives. This tendency of nature is not passive. One could never call it a mere wishful thinking. In point of fact, it is to a great degree the psychological basis for man's actions. He acts not only in order to live but also to satisfy the drive within himself to self-protection and development. One of

---

vitae ordinatur. Et ideo difficilius est vincere timorem periculorum mortis quam concupiscentiam delectationum, quae est in cibis et veneres." Ibid., q. 142, art. 3, ad 2.

[63] "Natura particularis est conservativa uniusquisque individui quantum potest; under praeter intentionem eius est quod deficiat in conservando." Ibid., q. 142, art. 3, ad 2.

[64] "Et secumdum hanc, omnis corruptio et defectus est contra naturam ... quia huiusmodi virtus intendit esse et conservationem eius cuis est." Ibid., I-II, q. 85, art. 6, in corp.

[65] "Actus igitur huiusmodi ex hoc quod intenditur conservatio propriae vitae, non habet rationem illiciti: cum hoc sit cuilibet naturale quod se conservet in esse quantum potest." Ibid., II-II, q. 64, art. 7, in corp.

the demands of nature, then, is the conservation of one's own life. Since it is true that man is bound to live according to his nature, it is also true to say that man is bound by the law of nature to conserve his own life.

This argument is based not on the presence or apparent absence of this natural inclination within a particular man. Rather, it is based on the presence of this inclination in an individual as is observed in the majority of mankind. The objection, therefore, that a man could easily fancy his self-development as existing in some form of suicide, in no way vitiates the argument. Reasoning in argumentation of this type should be grounded on the solid manifestations of the feelings and actions of mankind in general, not on the psychological quirks of any particular individual.

A review, therefore, of the foregoing discussions indicates that neither Scripture, the tradition of the teaching Church, nor the nature of man can be cited in support of an argument denying the obligation to conserve one's life. Indeed, the facts reveal the contrary. The reasons demonstrating the malice of suicide and the obligation of self-conservation are intimately related, and the common Catholic teaching has been consistent and constant in regard to both.

The teachings of Sacred Scripture and of the Church in this matter are merely authoritative restatements of what is already contained in the natural law.[66] Therefore, throughout this dissertation the malice of suicide is condemned as a grave infraction of the natural law, and the obligation of self-conservation is urged as a positive precept of the natural law—the supposition being that the reader in both instances will advert to the fact that the natural law is the foundation for any teaching in these matters found in Scripture or the

---

[66] In this dissertation, the natural law is understood as the natural *moral* law, as distinct from the physical laws of nature.

teaching of the Church. This applies also to man's natural inclination to conserve his life. Such an inclination manifests the content of the natural law for an individual in regard to the conservation of his life. The natural law in this matter, as in all others, is consonant with the very nature of man. Therefore, not to conserve one's life or, in effect, to commit suicide directly is entirely against nature and therefore intrinsically wrong.

Euthanasia and the Precept of Self-conservation

In the light of the foregoing arguments, a condemnation of euthanasia presents no problem. If euthanasia is inflicted without the consent of the patient, then it is intrinsically evil because it is murder. (The malice of homicide is treated elsewhere in the texts of Catholic moral theology.) If on the other hand, it is a form of voluntary euthanasia in which the person concerned gives permission on his own authority for his life to be taken, then it still remains intrinsically evil. The reason is a simple corollary to the discussions already made in this dissertation. Voluntary euthanasia is suicide and, as such, is a grave disregard of the obligation of self-conservation.

Epikeia

A question can easily arise which fittingly calls for attention here. Is it possible to apply *epikeia* to the natural law? More precisely, understanding *epikeia* as a correction of a law made by the subject himself on the presumption that the legislator did not intend to include his particular case in the law,[67] is it possible to apply *epikeia* in the question of

---

[67] L. Riley, *The History, Nature and Use of Epikeia in Moral Theology* (Washington, D.C.: Catholic University of America Press, 1948), p. 137.

the demand of the natural law that a man must not commit suicide and that he must conserve his life?

We must reply that there can never be an application of *epikeia* to the natural law and, therefore, not even in this case. In a thorough treatment of *epikeia*, Father Lawrence Riley devotes an entire chapter of his doctoral dissertation (1948) to this subject.[68] In this chapter the author assigns the many reasons in support of this doctrine. First of all, since the acts prescribed by the natural law are intrinsically good, and those forbidden are intrinsically evil, any possible extrinsic circumstances could never legitimately excuse an individual from positing the prescribed acts continuously or from avoiding, as a rule, the prohibited actions.[69] Furthermore, presuming that the licit use of *epikeia* is conditioned on the existence of the fact that the law is deficient, there can be no licit application of *epikeia* in the question of the natural law because there can be no defect in the Legislator, God; the promulgator, right reason; or the matter of the law, because it comprises what is either intrinsically good or intrinsically evil.[70] Therefore, whether the precepts of the natural law are negative or affirmative, the conclusion is that the natural law never admits of *epikeia*. An example of a negative precept of the natural law is the prohibition of suicide; an affirmative precept would be the duty of self-conservation. The following lines from Riley's work, which are based on the teaching of Suarez, are of considerable interest:

> For the negative precepts bind *semper* and *pro semper*, and hence the obligation can never cease. The affirmative precepts bind *semper* but not *pro semper*. Natural reason or positive law dictates when

---

[68] Ibid., pp. 258–291.
[69] Ibid., p. 277.
[70] Ibid., pp. 280–282.

precisely they must be put into execution. Not to fulfill them in *actu secundo* when, in the judgment of natural reason such is not demanded, is certainly no example of *epikeia*—it is simply an instance of interpretation. On the other hand, there can be no licit use of *epikeia* when reason dictates that the affirmative precepts of the natural law must be put into action. For to allow *epikeia* in such an instance would be to permit an action admittedly contrary to right reason and ultimately to the Divine Essence.[71]

Hence, since *epikeia* can never be licitly applied to the natural law,[72] the further deduction is true: namely, *epikeia* could never be employed by any individual on the grounds that his particular circumstances represent a case where the natural law would not require the fulfillment of the obligation of self-conservation.

Dispensation

A further question comes to mind. Is there such a thing as a dispensation from the natural law? Again, more precisely, can one obtain a dispensation from the obligation of conserving his life?

Dispensation is defined as the relaxation of a law in a particular case.[73] The natural law is by its very nature immu-

---

[71] Ibid., pp. 284–285.

[72] Further references to the question of epikeia and the natural law include Aertnys-Damen, *Theologiae moralis*, I, p. 126, quaer. 3; and Fanfani, *Manuale theorico-practicum theologiae moralis*, I, p. 19, dub. II. Fanfani explains that the application of epikeia to the natural law is impossible, because the natural law in founded in the very nature of man and comes from the supreme and most wise Legislator, and thus the law cannot be deficient, neither can there be a particular case not forseen by the omniscient Legislator.

[73] *Code of Canon Law* (1983), can. 85.

table and universal. Hence, there can be no dispensation from it. Since the natural law is immutable, it cannot be either suspended or abrogated, and since it is universal, it admits of no exception.[74] However, a certain type of mutability in the improper sense is admitted by some authors regarding the secondary precepts of the natural law.[75] They distinguish between the changing of a law and the changing of the matter of a law. Thus, a law properly could be called mutable if the obligation of the law ceases while at the same time the very same matter is involved. On the other hand, it would be called a mutable law in the improper sense if the obligation of the law ceases because the matter of the law has changed. The matter of the law here is understood as the item concerning which a law is formed and promulgated. Hence, these authors would say that regarding the secondary precepts, the natural law is mutable, in the improper sense, in a situation where the matter of the law has changed. Wherefore, a proper authority can dispense from the natural law in such a situation unless the law concerns a matter in itself everywhere and always intrinsically evil.

Others deny any type of mutation whatever in the natural law, as long as the demands of the law are expressed in complete and adequate terms with all the necessary restrictions, conditions, and determinations which would allow the applications of the law not only in general cases but also in particular and extraordinary cases.[76] Hence, these authors

---

[74] Fanfani, *Manuale theorico-practicum theologiae moralis*, I, p. 196.

[75] See Noldin-Schmitt, *Summa theologiae moralis*, I, p. 123, n. 116; Aertnys-Damen, *Theologiae moralis*, I, p. 125, n. 136; Lehmkuhl, *Theologia moralis*, I, p. 122; and Fanfani, *Manuale theorico-practicum theologiae moralis*, I, pp. 196–197.

[76] Regatillo-Zalba, *Theologiae moralis summa*, I, p. 354.

feel there is no possible dispensation from the natural law, because, as is known, the indispensability of the natural law derives from its immutability. Therefore, they would say that there is no dispensation from the natural law, even in the improper sense. Any cases which are brought forth as examples of a dispensation from the natural law merely manifest special conditions which do not permit the application of a principle of the natural law because it has been expressed in terms too general and indefinite.[77]

Whatever remains to be said of this dispute would not be to the point here. Perhaps the whole matter represents merely an argument over words, because all admit that the natural law in itself is immutable and admits of no dispensation in that sense.

Therefore, an individual can never receive a dispensation from the obligation of conserving his life. God could manifest His will and demand that a person give up his life by some form of non-conservation of self. This would not be a divine dispensation from the natural law. God has the dominion over life, and He can cede this faculty to man, and thus the non-conservation of self or suicide would not be against the natural law, since the individual would be acting not on his own authority but on God's. Killing is not against the natural law; it is killing without the proper authority that breaks the natural law. This authority is not a dispensation, not a jurisdictional act whereby the natural law is relaxed in a particular case; rather, it is a divine permission to exercise a faculty which God ordinarily reserves to Himself. In passing, it should be noted that an individual must have positive evidence that this faculty has been granted him by God. Presumption, instigated by the onslaught of physical or psychological ills, is certainly no indication that God has given such a faculty.

---

[77] Ibid., pp. 355–356.

Ignorance

Another interesting point is the possibility of invincible ignorance in this matter. In effect, the question is, Can there be invincible ignorance of the natural law, or, rather, is the natural law so well written and impressed in the hearts of men that it is quite inconceivable that a man could be invincibly ignorant of its demands? Certainly, one of the basic postulates of the natural law is the precept of self-conservation. This is grounded on a very natural inclination. It would seem, therefore, that no possibility of invincible ignorance in this matter could ever be present.

In point of fact, the history of the world and of different races testifies that it has been with considerable difficulty that some peoples have arrived at the knowledge of even the most fundamental moral truths. It is also true that in the present condition of fallen nature, the promulgation of the natural law by the light of the human reason alone is sufficient physically for a man to know the content of the natural law. However, human reason alone is insufficient morally—hence the need of revelation. In fact, divine revelation in this present economy is morally necessary in order that the natural law can be known with sufficient ease, certitude, and completeness.[78]

The common teaching holds that an individual enjoying the use of reason cannot be in ignorance of the first and most universal principles of the natural law.[79] Furthermore, the primary conclusions drawn from the most universal principles are also known, and the individual cannot be invincibly ignorant of these for any extended length of time,

---

[78] A. Vermeersch, *Theologiae moralis principia-responsa-consilia*, I, p. 127.

[79] Regatillo-Zalba, *Theologiae moralis summa*, I, p. 361, n. 344; Fanfani, *Manuale theorico-practicum theologiae moralis*, p. 198.

because the ordinary intellect can deduce these conclusions correctly with a minimum of effort. The foregoing, then, is the common teaching regarding the knowledge that a human being has of the natural law. However, it is necessary to admit that defects of education, past sins and evil habits, and false persuasions can be the cause of invincible ignorance for a time.[80]

Vincible ignorance, which is also culpable, obviously can be present, not because of a defect in the intellect but due to a bad will—with this point there is no argument.[81] Over and above this, there can also be a situation in which the intellect would draw the correct conclusion from a most universal principle but err in the application of the conclusion to a particular case.[82]

It is necessary, then, to admit theoretically first of all that cases of invincible ignorance of the natural law can occur, and therefore the person concerned is free of the guilt of formal sin. The opposite opinion, once held by the Jansenists, was condemned in 1690 by Pope Alexander VIII:

> Although there may be invincible ignorance of the law of nature, in the state of fallen nature, the one working in virtue of this ignorance is not excused from sin.[83]

---

[80]Regatillo-Zalba, *Theologiae moralis summa*, I, n. 345; Fanfani, *Manuale theorico-practicum theologiae moralis*, p. 199.

[81]Noldin-Schmitt, *Summa theologiae moralis*, I, p. 122, n. 144.

[82]Regatillo-Zalba, *Theologiae moralis summa*, I, p. 362 note 48.

[83]"Tametsi detur ignorantia invicibilis iuris naturae, haec in statu naturae lapsae operantem ex ipsa non excusat a peccato formali." Decree of the Holy Office, December 7, 1690, Denzinger 1292.

Secondly, one has to agree that an individual can err in good faith in the application of a natural law principle or deduction and thus, also, be free of guilt.

Now to the case in point. The principle guiding an individual to the conservation of his life is self-evident. *Per se*, therefore, there can be no invincible ignorance in this regard. The drive leading a man forward to self-conservation finds its roots in the very nature of man. He cannot be ignorant for any extended length of time of the obligation of self-conservation. However, the following would seem to be possibilities:

1. Theoretically, an individual, for a brief time, could be invincibly ignorant of the duty of self-conservation. Thus he would not be guilty of sin if in that period of time, and acting in virtue of the invincible ignorance, he should take his life.

2. A situation can occur in which an individual would be vincibly and culpably ignorant of his obligation of self-conversation. Any action performed in virtue of this ignorance would, of course, be sinful.

3. An individual could fully realize his obligation to self-conservation and admit its truth but feel that his failure to satisfy the obligation would be licit because of some particular circumstances. A good example of this is euthanasia. The patient could falsely justify euthanasia because of the overwhelming pain he is suffering. The doctor could falsely justify his administration of the euthanasia on the grounds of charity to the patient. This is ignorance not regarding the law itself but rather regarding the application of the law, and thus again an individual might escape formal sin:

> However it was conceded that *per accidens* the subject may conceive an action as justifiable in practical action surrounded with all its circumstances while fully admitting the general prohibition. This would hold in the present consideration. The aversion to

the physical pain that causes men to subvert the value of life to the value of physical well-being is no doubt due to a long series of sins on the part of both individuals and society. However, as has been seen, ignorance which is a consequence of sin is not always culpable ignorance. If it is a result of previous sin, it is not culpable unless it had been foreseen. Though its admission constitutes an indictment of modern society, the possibility of invincible ignorance of the evil of euthanasia is to be admitted. The same principles can sometimes be applied to suicide.[84]

One must enjoy the use of reason before the above-mentioned rules on ignorance of the natural law apply. This does not mean, of course, that those who have not as yet reached the use of reason and those who are insane are not bound by the natural law. Rather, the opposite obtains. These people, like all other human beings, by their very nature are subject to the natural law, and thus when they break this law, they sin—materially, however, and not formally.[85]

Principle of the Double Effect

The principle of the double effect also comes to mind, and a question arises concerning it. Can the principle of the double effect be used in certain cases involving the dictate of the natural law requiring self-conservation? Is it licit to perform some action which will produce two effects—one of which will be an individual's own death? Up till now, therefore, the discussion has centered on the necessity of self-conservation and the malice of non-conservation of

---

[84] S. Bertke, *The Possibility of Invincible Ignorance of the Natural Law* (Washington, D.C.: Catholic University Press, 1941), p. 103.

[85] See Aertnys-Damen, *Theologiae moralis*, I, p. 124.

self by some form of direct suicide. Here, the question of indirect suicide comes into light.

Obviously, any form of non-conservation of self that happens without any intention at all on the part of the individual is without fault. It then is involuntary as, for example, in the case of an accidental suicide. However, in the case of an action which is entirely intended and willed but which will produce two effects, one of which is good and the other evil, it would be licit to perform this action only if certain conditions are fulfilled. Father Edwin Healy, S.J., explains it this way:

> It is allowable to actuate a cause that will produce a good and bad effect, provided (1) the good effect and not the evil effect is directly intended; (2) the action itself is good, or at least, indifferent; (3) the good effect is not produced by means of the evil effect; and (4) there is a proportionate reason for permitting the foreseen evil effect to occur.[86]

Above all, it is necessary to underline the fact that, just as direct suicide performed on one's own authority is always illicit, so also indirect suicide which is not accompanied by a proportionately grave reason is basically illicit. Indirect suicide is understood here as suicide eventuating from the performance or omission of an act on account of which death occurs. The moral difference in the two forms of suicide lies in the fact that indirect suicide can sometimes be licit if there is a proportionately grave reason on account of which the indirect suicide can be permitted.

Hence, the application of all the above principles to particular cases would show that the following solutions

---

[86] E. Healy, *Moral Guidance* (Chicago: Loyola University Press, 1942), p. 20.

offered by the older moralists are valid.[87] (1) A soldier may remain at his post even though he is morally certain that he will be killed. (2) An individual in a shipwreck may give his means of safety to someone else, even though the loss of his own life may occur. (3) One may minister to those infected with contagious fatal diseases even with great danger to his own life. (4) In the event of a fire, it is licit to jump from a high position with the intention of escaping the fire even though there is certain danger of death involved in such a high fall. Likewise, a young woman could do the same in order to escape an attacker. (5) Naval personnel could scuttle a ship at sea during war even with danger and possible death occurring to themselves, lest the enemy capture the ship and thus inflict heavy damage on their native land. (6) It is also licit to fast and abstain and inflict moderate injuries on one's body for the sake of penance, even though, unintentionally, one's span of life is considerably shortened.

Certainly, these cases are not the only ones possible to mention. The principles involved are clear. With the examples that have been given, the distinction between direct and indirect non-conservation of self has been sufficiently outlined.

There is an interesting case, however, which is worthy of separate mention, because there could be a serious temptation to solve the problem by means of the two-fold effect principle. This, however, would seem to be unlawful and not allowable. These days, an episode involving voluntary hunger strike occasionally occurs. As a rule, it receives tremendous publicity in the ordinary daily journals. This is true

---

[87] The following examples are from Alphonsus, *Theologica moralis*, lib. III, tract. 4, cap. I, dub. 1, nn. 366, 367, and 371. They are also given in his *Homo apostolicus* (Turin: Marietti, 1848), tract. VIII, cap. 1, n. 1.

especially when the ones involved undertake their hunger strike in order to emphasize or solve some public issue. The fascinating story of the voluntary hunger strike of the Lord Mayor of Cork, Ireland, in 1920 is typical. This gentleman, in order to defend the autonomy of Ireland against England, had recourse to a voluntary hunger strike and died on October 25, 1920, after a fast from food which lasted seventy-three days, twelve hours, and forty minutes.[88]

It is quite simple to imagine that many, especially those emotionally connected with the situation, could fancy that some species of the principle of the double effect would justify the actual non-conservation of self on the part of the famous mayor of Cork. There were, no doubt, several who felt at the time that the autonomy of the country, the striving after a great good, and the interest in the common weal made his course of action licit.

An examination of the case proves, of course, that only a valid application of the two-fold effect principle could justify the situation. Certainly, the bare action alone of the mayor was not allowable, because it was direct non-conservation of self. However, a thorough analysis reveals that no application of the principle of the double effect would seem to be allowable here. The act of fasting is certainly good or, at least, indifferent. The good effect, namely, the recognition of Ireland's autonomy, was what was directly intended, and certainly the bad effect was not the means by which the good effect would come. However, it would seem that this particular hunger strike was not allowable. Although the act of fasting in the beginning was good or at least indifferent morally, the point eventually came when fasting ceased being a morally indifferent act. As the mayor's physical condition

---

[88] See editor's note in *La Documentation Catholique*, October 30, 1920, p. 333.

became worse, then fasting any longer became unlawful because of the grave injury to health and the danger of death involved. Furthermore, whether the action in itself were good or not, it certainly was an inefficacious means of obtaining the end in view. Thus, the mayor's action should be condemned also on the grounds of lacking a proportionately grave reason. It is difficult to agree that a voluntary hunger-strike on the part of the mayor of Cork would be a secure means, efficacious by its very nature, and the only means necessary and proportioned to the obtaining of national liberty and independence.[89]

This case is cited here to show, first of all, an example of an invalid application of the principle of the double effect, and also to emphasize that even when suicide is not directly intended, a voluntary and direct abstinence from food, complete and lasting till death, even though performed because of high political or social motives, remains illicit nonetheless.[90] It can be said, in passing, that the mayor of Cork acted in good faith and thus was free from formal sin.

Thus far, the treatment of cases involving non-conservation of one's life has involved, first of all, direct suicide, and this is always illicit. Secondly, the possibilities of indirect suicide were mentioned together with stipulated reasons and conditions because of which the indirect suicide could be allowable. In the first of these cases, the non-conservation of self is said to be voluntary and thus sinful. In the second, it is not voluntary but is said to be permitted, and thus can, at times, be licit if certain conditions are verified.

---

[89] *La Civiltà Cattolica*, IV (1920), pp. 530–531. See also P. Gannon, "La Grève de la Faim," *La Documentation Catholique* 30 (1920), pp. 333–336; and *L'Ami du Clergé* (1920), pp. 529ss.

[90] See Aertnys-Damen, *Theologiae moralis*, I, p. 457 note 1.

Thirdly, the case of the completely accidental, unforeseen non-conservation of self was mentioned. This is entirely involuntary, and therefore free of any moral culpability. In all three of these cases, though, the common element is some positive action performed by the individual which directly or indirectly brings about his death. There is present, therefore, a cause which exerts a positive influence in the matter.

Moral Impossibility

Now what about a mere omission of an action, when by this omission death of one's self occurs? Would it be illicit for an individual to omit an action when he foresees that he could perform the action and that, should he choose not to, he will die? (Furthermore, the supposition in the case would be that he really would not intend to choose death, or else, of course, it would be suicide.)

In treating the famous Cork case, we mentioned actually a situation involving the omission of food. However, at the time, the point of main concern was an explanation of the conditions involved in the licit application of the two-fold effect principle. Here our main concern is the direct treatment of the principles involved in the omission of an act. The reason for the separate mention of the moral principles involved in this question is the fact that they are of great importance in determining the obligation that an individual has of conserving his life in certain circumstances. We shall see the application of these principles more clearly as this dissertation progresses.

Three conditions are necessary in order that a person be charged with guilt in a situation which involves either the omission of an act in impeding evil or the placing of an act which causes evil, even though the effects of evil are not intended: (1) In some manner, at least in a confused way, he must foresee the evil effect. (2) He must be able to prevent the evil either by acting or omitting an action. (3) He must be bound by some obligation to prevent the evil.[91]

In the case at hand, therefore, the supposition is that an individual can perform the action and that he foresees that if he does not, he will die; he does not, however, intend his death. Therefore, the response is that he is guilty of sin if he omits the conservation of his life, unless it should be in his case that he (this particular individual) is not bound to conserve his life. Yet, on the other hand, it is a dictate of the natural law that a person conserve his life.

When does the moral obligation of the natural law cease? The answer to this question is quite simple. The obligation imposed by the natural law never ceases. It binds every human being, everywhere and always. However, it is possible that a human individual could be excused from the fulfillment of the natural law because of particular circumstances. One of the excusing causes is ignorance of the law. This has been treated earlier. Another, however, is inability to fulfill the law. This inability can be of a physical nature. Certainly, no one is bound morally to fulfill a law when he is physically unfit to do so. This is obvious in the question of the conservation of one's own life. Otherwise, an individual would be morally bound to the performance of the impossible, and this is a patent contradiction.[92] On the other hand, the individual may be physically capable of fulfilling the law but unable to, here and now, because of some circumstance of fear, danger, or grave inconvenience which renders the observance of the law extremely difficult for him. It is then said to be morally impossible for him to fulfill the law. It is obvious that physical inability excuses from the observance of a precept of the natural law. Regarding moral inability, however, the following

---

[91] Lehmkuhl, *Theologia moralis*, I, p. 20.
[92] See Denzinger 804.

is to be noted. Theologians commonly distinguish between the affirmative and negative precepts of the natural law.[93] In the case of the negative precepts, it is necessary to emphasize that they are always binding even when their fulfillment involves a grave danger of death. This is so because these negative precepts forbid what is intrinsically evil, and not even death itself would make it licit to perform evil. So no grave inconvenience would produce a moral impossibility in this regard.

Where an affirmative precept is concerned, however, a moral inability would excuse from the fulfillment or observance of the precept. The reason is that these laws bind an individual *semper* but not *pro semper*, as the common dictum puts it, whereas in the case of negative precepts, the obligation is *semper* and *pro semper*.[94] It is a rational presumption then that since man is not always and everywhere, under every circumstance, bound to do something positively good, he would not be always and everywhere bound to fulfill an affirmative precept. Hence, a moral impossibility, while not freeing an individual from the basic obligation of the natural law, excuses him from the present observance of an affirmative precept of that law.[95]

---

[93] Noldin-Schmitt, *Summa theologiae moralis*, I, p. 179, n. 177.

[94] See L. Fanfani, *Manuale theorico-practicum theologiae moralis*, I, p. 184 and p. 272; also Lehmkuhl, *Theologia moralis*, I, p. 108.

[95] There are occasions when an affirmative law binds even in the presence of moral impossibility: (1) if the violation of the law brings about common harm, (2) if the violation tends to the detriment of religion or hatred of God, (3) if the violation tends to the grave detriment of the spiritual condition of the individual concerned. See Lehmkuhl, *Theologia moralis*, I, pp. 108–109; and Noldin-Schmitt, *Summa theologiae moralis*, I, p. 179, par. 177, n. 2.

One further point worthy of note is the fact that an instance of moral impossibility does not exist in a situation where the fulfillment of the law is intrinsically and radically accompanied by some considerable inconvenience.[96] This is a difficulty common to all men and thus would not generally constitute a moral impossibility for any one individual. So, for example, the ordinary individual usually could not excuse himself from the obligation of obtaining food on the grounds that working for the money to buy the food constitutes for him a moral impossibility. In the case, however, where working would entail a difficulty for him not commonly experienced by men in general, then a possible instance of moral inability to fulfill the law might exist.

Therefore, to summarize the above doctrine and apply it to the problem at hand: an individual is always bound by the affirmative precept of the natural law commanding him to conserve his life. However, the individual is licitly excused from the fulfillment of this precept by circumstances which constitute for him a moral impossibility not commonly experienced by men in general. How grave this difficulty has to be is the question which will occupy a great section of the remainder of this dissertation.

Ordinary and Extraordinary Means

The law that demands the conservation of one's own life also commands that one employ the means necessary to conserve one's life. Since, however, this law is an affirmative law and a licit application of the doctrine on moral impossibility may be made, theologians commonly divide the means of conserving life into two categories. The first includes those which are obligatory for everyone. The second comprises those means whose use would constitute a moral

---

[96] Lehmkuhl, *Theologia moralis*, I.

impossibility either for human beings in general or for one particular individual. The former they term *ordinary means*, the latter *extraordinary means*. An individual must employ the ordinary means of conserving his life. *Per se*, he need not use the extraordinary means. *Per accidens*, however, someone might have the obligation of employing the means which are recognized as extraordinary for him and for human beings in general.

In this chapter, we have investigated the basic obligation that binds each individual to conserve his life. We have seen also that because this precept is affirmative, the individual is held *per se* to employ only the ordinary means of conserving his life, *per accidens* the extraordinary means. In the next chapter, we shall review the teaching of Catholic theologians regarding the nature and use of these ordinary and extraordinary means of conserving life.

CONCLUSIONS

1. God retains the radical possession of the rights over man's life. Man has full rights to the use of his life but to this only. Hence, any form of non-conservation of self, directly intended by an individual on his own authority, is illicit.

2. Likewise, man has the serious positive obligation of caring for his bodily life and health.

3. It is possible that an individual could be invincibly ignorant of this obligation for a time, but certainly not for any extended length of time. However, it is possible that one might realize his obligation to conserve his life but err in the practical application of the obligation to his status here and now.

4. There is no licit application of *epikeia* in this matter. Neither is a dispensation possible. However, an individual could receive the command from God to

take his own life by some form of non-conservation of self. In such a case, the individual would then have permission to exercise a faculty ordinarily reserved as a divine prerogative.

5. The obligation to conserve one's life, being an affirmative precept of the natural law, does not require fulfillment under all circumstances. Hence a moral impossibility would excuse.

6. The means to fulfill this precept of self-conservation are obligatory. Those means binding everyone in common circumstances are ordinary means. Those means involving a moral impossibility are extraordinary means.

Chapter 2

The History of Ordinary and Extraordinary Means

Inasmuch as the main object of this dissertation is an analysis of the Catholic teaching concerning the ordinary and extraordinary means of conserving life, it is fitting that, from the outset, a simple report of the traditional opinions on this subject be given. However, to conjoin an analysis with this report would be far too cumbersome. Hence, the reader will find that an attempt has been made to keep the commentary on the opinions cited here to a minimum. A more lengthy analysis will follow in the next chapter.

Thirteenth to Sixteenth Centuries

Having in mind the basic duty which obliges an individual to conserve his life, as was seen in the preceding chapter, we will now find it rather interesting to follow the further development of this doctrine through the centuries. The present historical report commences with St. Thomas Aquinas. In point of fact, there was not much discussion of the problem of the ordinary and extraordinary means of conserving life in the writings of the theologians prior to the sixteenth century. We begin with St. Thomas, however, because his treatment of the question of suicide in the

Summa theologica (II-II, q. 64, art. 5) influenced later writers quite heavily. Furthermore, many of the commentators chose this article[1] and the one on mutilation (II-II, q. 65, art. 1)[2] as the place for their discussion of the ordinary and extraordinary means of conserving life. Citations have already been given from St. Thomas. The following one, however, is of particular interest:

> A man has the obligation to sustain his body, otherwise he would be a killer of himself. ... By precept, therefore, he is bound to nourish his body, and likewise we are bound to all the other items without which the body cannot live.[3]

The theologians immediately succeeding St. Thomas were content merely to restate his arguments against suicide,[4] and one does not discover in their writings any lengthy speculation regarding the use of the ordinary and extraordinary means of conserving life.

SIXTEENTH TO LATE SEVENTEENTH CENTURIES

In the sixteenth century much discussion about the problem occurs. One of the notable theologians in this regard is Francisco de Vitoria, O.P. (1492–1546). In his famous *Relectiones theologiae*, there is much of considerable interest.

---

[1] See *Somme theologique*, II, *La justice*, p. 149.

[2] For example, see D. Bañez, *Scholastica commentaria in partem angelici doctoris S. Thomae* (Douai, 1614–1615), tom. IV, *Decisiones de iure et iustitia*, in II-II, q. 65, art. 1.

[3] "Praecipitur autem homini quod corpus suum sustentet, alias, enim est homicida ipsius ... ex praecepto ergo tenetur homo corpus suum nutrire et similiter ad omnia sine quibus corpus non potest vivere, tenemur." Thomas Aquinas, *Super epistolas S. Pauli* (Turin: Marietti, 1953), II Thess., lec. 11, n. 77.

[4] See, for example, Antonius, *Theologica moralis* (Verona, 1740), *De homicidio*, tom. II, col. 861, lit. D.

This holds true of his commentary on the *Secunda Secundae* of St. Thomas also. First of all, in the *Relectio de temperantia*, Vitoria treats many problems regarding one's life by means of food. He proves this obligation by arguments based on man's natural inclination to self-conservation, the love a man owes himself and the malice of suicide contained in the non-conservation of self. Therefore, if the conservation of self by food is an obligation, it would seem that a sick person who did not eat because of some disgust for food would be guilty of mortal sin. Vitoria replies,

> Regarding the first argument to the contrary, ...
> I would say secondly that if a sick man can take
> food or nourishment with some hope of life, he is
> held to take the food, as he would be held to give it
> to one who is sick. Thirdly, I would say that if the
> depression of spirit is so low and there is present
> such consternation in the appetitive power that only
> with the greatest of effort and as though by means
> of a certain torture can the sick man take food, right
> away that is reckoned a certain impossibility, and
> therefore he is excused, at least from mortal sin,
> especially where there is little hope of life or none
> at all. Responding by way of confirmation: first of
> all a similar case does not exist in reference to food
> and drugs. For food is *per se* a means ordered to the
> life of the animal and it is natural, drugs are not:
> man is not held to employ all the possible means of
> conserving his life, but the means which are *per se*
> intended for that purpose. ... Thirdly, we say that
> if one were to have moral certitude that by means
> of a drug he would gain health, without the drug,
> however, he would die, he really does not seem to be
> excused from mortal sin: because if he did not give
> the drug to a sick neighbor, he would sin mortally,
> and medicine *per se* is intended also by nature for
> health, but since this rarely can be certain, therefore
> they are not to be condemned of mortal sin who
> have universally declared an abstinence from drugs,

although this is not laudable because God created medicine because of its need, as Solomon says. [5]

Later, then, discussing the lawfulness of abstaining perpetually from a certain type of food, even in extreme necessity, Vitoria has this to say:

> Finally, for a solution of the objections, it must be noted: it is one thing not to protect life and it is another to destroy it: for man is not always held to the first and it is enough that he perform that by which regularly a man can live: if a sick man could not have a drug except by giving over his whole means of subsistence, I do not think he would be bound to do so.[6]

---

[5] "Ad argumentum in contrarium, ad primum. ... Secundo dico quod si aegrotus potest semere cibum, vel alimentum cum aliqua spe vitae, tenetur sumere cibum, sicut teneretur dare aegrotanti. Tertio dico, quod si animi dejectio tanta est et appetitivae virtutis tanta consternatio, ut non nisi per summum laborem et quasi cruciatum quendam, aegrotus possit sumere cibum, jam reputatur quaedam impossibilitas et ideo exclusatur, saltem a mortali, maxime ubi est exigua spes vitae aut nulla. Ad confirmationem respondetur. Primo, quod non est simile de pharmaco et alimento. Alimentum enim per se ad hoc ordinatum ad vitam animalis est naturale, non autem pharmacum: nec tenetur homo adhibere, omnia media possibilia ad conservandam vitam, sed media per se ad hoc ordinata. ... Tertio dicimus quod si quis haberet certitudinem moraliter, quod per pharmacum reciperet incolumitatem, sine pharmaco autem moreretur, noon videtur profecto excusari a mortali: quia si non daret pharmacam proximo sic aegrotanti, peccaret mortaliter et medicina per se etiam ordinata est ad salutem a natura, sed quia hoc xiv potest esse certum, ideo non sunt damnandi de mortali, qui in universum decreverunt abstinere a pharmacis, licet non sit laudabile, cum creaverit Deus medicinam propter necessitatem ut aid Salomon." F. de Vitoria, *Relectiones theologicae* (Lyon, 1587), relectio IX, *De temperantia*, n. 1.

[6] "Pro solutione tandem argumentorum, notandum est: quod aliud est non protelare vitam, aliud est abrumpere: nam ad

Then he adds,

> Second conclusion: One is not held to protect his
> life as much as he can by means of foods. This is
> clear because one is not held to use foods which are
> the best, the most delicate and most expensive, even
> though these foods are the most healthful; indeed,
> this is blameworthy. ... Likewise, one is not held
> to live in the most healthful place, therefore neither
> must he use the most healthful food.[7]

Again:

> Third conclusion: If one uses foods which men com-
> monly use and in the quantity which customarily
> suffices for the conservation of strength, even though
> from this his life is shortened, even notably and this
> is noticed, he would not sin. ... From this, the cor-
> ollary follows that one is not held to use medicines
> to prolong his life even where the danger of death is
> probable, for example to take for some years a drug
> to avoid fevers or anything of this sort.[8]

---

primum non semper tenetur homo et satis est, quod det operam,
per quam homo regulariter potest vivere: nec puto, si aeger non
posset habere pharmacum nisi daret totam substantiam suam,
quod teneretur facere." Ibid., n. 9.

[7] "Secunda conclusion: non tenetur quis protelare vitam per
alimenta quantum potest. Patet, quia non tenetur uti cibis optimus
et delicatissimis et pretoisissimis etiamsi ea sint saluberrima, imo
hoc est reprehensible. ... Item non tentur vivere in loco saluberrimo, ergo nec uti cibo saluberrimo." Ibid., n. 12.

[8] "Tertia conclusio: Si quis utatur alimentis, quibus homines communiter utuntur et in quantitate, quae solet sufficere
ad valetudinem conservandam, dato quod ex hoc abbrevietur
vita, etiam notabiliter et hoc percipiatur, non peccat. ... Ex quo
sequitur corollarium, quod non tenetur quis uti medicines, ad
prolongandum vitam, etiam ubi esset probabile periculum mortis, puta quotannis sumere pharmacum ad vitandas febrew, vela
aliquid huiusmodi." Ibid.

Another pertinent passage comes from Vitoria's *Relectio de homicidio*:

> One is not held, as I said, to employ all the means to conserve his life, but it is sufficient to employ the means which are of themselves intended for this purpose and congruent. Wherefore, in the case which has been posited, I believe that the individual is not held to give his whole inheritance to preserve his life. ... From this also it is inferred that when one is sick without hope of life, granted that a certain precious drug could produce life for some hours or even days, he would not be held to buy it, but it is sufficient to use common remedies, and he is considered as though dead.[9]

Vitoria uses the same reasoning in his commentary on St. Thomas:

> In the second place, I say that one is not held to lengthen his life, because he is not held to use always the most delicate foods, that is, hens and chickens, even though he has the ability and the doctors say that if he eats in such a manner, he will live twenty years more, and even if he knew this for certain, he would not be obliged. ... So I say, thirdly, that it is licit to eat common and regular foods. ... Granted that the doctor advises him to eat chickens and partridges, he can eat eggs and other common items.[10]

----

[9] "Non tenetur quis cti dixi, omnia media ponere ad servandum vitam, sed satis est ponere media ad hoc de se ordinate et congruentia. Unde in casu posito credo quod non tenetur dare totem patrimonium pro vita servanda. ... Ex quo etiam infertur, quod cum aliquis sine spe vitae aegrotat, dato quod aliquo pharmaco pretioso posset producere vitam aliquot horas, aut etiam dies, non tenetur illud emere, sed satis erit uti remediis communibus et ille reputatur quasi mortuus." Ibid., relectio X, *De homicidio*, n. 35.

[10] "Secundum dico non tenetur aliquis augere vitam quia non tenetur semper uti delicatissimus cibis, scilicet gallinis et pullus,

Finally:

> Where, however, one were to live in a very strict and
> singular manner, for example, eating perpetually
> only bread and water so that he abbreviates his life,
> perhaps it would not be licit, or even to eat only
> once in the week would not be licit. But this ought
> to happen in a manner common to good men so
> that it is beside one's intention that death follow
> and not by intention.[11]

Domingo de Soto, O.P. (1494–1560), in his *Theologia
moralis*, adheres to St. Thomas closely. Treating of suicide,[12]
he explicitly repeats the arguments of the Angelic Doctor.
Soto includes this treatment in his tract *De justitia et jure*.
The next point for explanation is the problem of mutilation. Soto, in this particular question, not only treats the
lawfulness and unlawfulness of mutilation but touches also
on the intriguing speculation of whether or not a person is
ever bound to suffer a mutilation and, further, whether the
individual could ever be forced to submit to a mutilation.
In the course of his discussion, Soto writes,

---

etiamsi habeat facultatem et medici dicant quod si comedit ex illis
vivet plus viginti annos et etiamsi hoc sciret pro certo, non tenetur. ... Et sic dico tertio, quod licet comedere cibos communes et
regulares. ... Dato quod medicus consuleret illi comedere pullos
et perdices, potest comedere ova et alia communia." F. de Vitoria,
Comentarios a la secunda secundae de Santo Tomas (Salamanca,
1932–1952), in II-II, q. 147, art. 1.

[11] "Ubi tamen modo arctissimo et singulari quis viveret,
puta non comendendo perpetuo nisi panem et aquam ut vitam
abbreviaret, forte non liceret vel etiam semel tantum in heb-
domada comedere non liceret. Sed debet hoc fieri modo communi
hominum bonorum ut preatur intentionem mors sequatur, et non
ex intentione." Ibid., q. 64, art. 1.

[12] Soto, *De justitia et jure*, lib. V, q. 1, art. 5.

A prelate indeed could force a subject, on account of a singular obedience promised to him, to take medicines which he can conveniently accept. But, really, no one can be forced to bear the tremendous pain in the amputation of a member or in an incision into the body: because no one is held to preserve his life with such torture. Neither is he thought to be the killer of himself.[13]

In his *De justitia commutativa*, Molina gives a good treatment of the status of man as the custodian and guardian of his life and members. In the course of this treatment he describes the necessity *"per accidens"* of using the extraordinary means of conserving life. The section has these words:

Fourth conclusion. Because man has been constituted the custodian and administrator of his own life and members, when he is unwilling, no one can cut a member from him for the sake of curing him or apply any other medicinal remedy to him.[14]

Soon again then, he says,

The conclusion proposed, therefore, is understood only when it is not entirely certain that the remedy will be of profit for avoiding the grave harm of a neighbor: or when the remedy is such that because of too intense a pain or another legitimate reason,

---

[13] "Praelatus vero cogere posset subditum propter singularem obedientiam illi promissam, ut medicamina admittat quae commode recipere potest. At vero quod ingentissimum dolorem in amputatione membri aut corporis incisione ferat, profecto nemo cogi potest: quia nemo tenetur tanto cruciatu vitam servare. Neque ille censendus est sui homocida." Ibid., q. 2, art. 1.

[14] "Quarta conclusio. Quia homo custos et administrator est constitutus suae propriae vitae ac membrorum, nullus ipso renuente, potest secare ad eo membrum gratia curationis, aut medicamentum aliud ei applicare." Molina, *De justitia et jure*, tom. IV, tract. III, disp 1, col. 514.

he is not obliged to undergo that which he needs in order to conserve his life or member.[15]

In this particular subject, namely, the necessity of using the ordinary means of conserving life and the lawfulness of shunning the extraordinary means, the teaching of Vitoria had tremendous influence.[16] Many of the authors used his speculation as the foundation for their own thinking in the matter. Others were quite content with repeating verbatim his doctrine. An example of this latter approach is found in the writing of Gregory Sayrus, O.S.B. (1560–1602). His famous *Clavis regia casuum conscientiae* contains in the ninth chapter of the seventh book much of what has already been cited from Vitoria. For instance, in the question of the lawfulness of abstinence from food and of penances administered to the body when such procedures injure one's health or shorten one's life, Sayrus uses the very arguments and words of Vitoria. Thus, one finds that he emphasizes that an individual is not bound to prolong his life,[17] nor

---

[15] "Conclusio ergo proposita solum intelligitur, quandon certum omnio non est remedium profuturum ad grave malum proximi, vitandum: aut quando omnio non est remedium profuturum ad grave malum proximi, vitandum: aut quando remedium est tale quod propter nimium dolorem, vel alia legitima causa, non tenetur is sub reatu lethalis culpae illud subire, qui eo indiget ad vitam aud membrum conservandum." Ibid.

[16] The influence of Vitoria is recognized not only in regard to this problem but also in regard to many other aspects of moral theology. "Vitoria fama celebratus ob suas Relectiones, in quibus, derelinquens sentias Lombardi, felici innovationae a posteris imitanda sollerter Summam Aquintis commentatus est, cum applicationibus ad quaestiones novas sui temporis." Regatillo-Zalba, *Theologiae moralis summa*, I, p. 25.

[17] G. Sayrus, *Clavis regia casuum conscientae* (Venice, 1625), lib. VII, cap. IX, n. 28.

is one held to use the very best and more delicate foods.[18]
However, Sayrus adds to the expression "common foods"
the notion of their being produced naturally:

> No one in order to prolong his life is bound to use
> the best and more delicate foods, even though he
> can, but the common ones, naturally produced.[19]

Later, he expresses in his own words an idea also found in
Vitoria:

> For although a man is held not to cut off his life,
> he is not held, however, to seek all the means, even
> licit ones, in order to make his life longer. This is
> manifest because, granted that an individual should
> know for certain that in India or in another city,
> even nearby, the air is more healthful and milder and
> that there he would live longer than in his native
> land or in his own city, he is not bound, however,
> to seek all the means, even licit and exquisite ones,
> in order to make his life longer.[20]

Again Sayrus repeats the teaching of Vitoria cited earlier
in this chapter regarding the use of medicine,[21] after which
he says, "Not all means must be furnished for the sake of
conserving life, but those only which for this purpose are

---

[18] Ibid.

[19] "Nemo ad vitam prolongandam, cibis optimus et delicatioribus uti tenetur, etiamsi possit, sed communibus naturaliter
productis." Ibid.

[20] "Quamvis enim teneatur homo non abrumpere vitam non
tenetur tamen omnia media etiam licita et exquisite quaerere,
ut longiorem vitam faciat. Id quod manifeste patet, quia dato,
quod aliquis certo sciat, quod in India aut in alia civitate etiam
propinqua salubrior et clementior aura sit et quod ibi diutius
viveret, quam in patria, aut propia civitate, non tenetur tamen
omnia media etiam licita et exquisita quaerere ut longiorem vitam
faciat." Ibid.

[21] Ibid.

necessary and congruous."[22] Finally, Sayrus reaches the problem of mutilation and answers the question whether or not, when a sick person is unwilling, he may be forced as a citizen by the state, as a son by his father, or as a subject by a prelate to submit to the mutilation of one of his members. Sayrus shows himself indebted to Soto in his answer. His general response is in the affirmative if the person is necessary for the common good.

If the mutilation, however, is necessary only for the particular good and health of the sick individual, then he cannot be forced. To this he adds,

> Furthermore, since by the natural law each one is bound to employ for the conservation of his body those licit means which he can conveniently undertake, the individual undoubtedly would sin who, when there is no question of great pain, would permit himself to die when he could take care of the health of his body. To this, however, that he suffer the very intense pain of the amputation of a member or of an incision into his body, neither a prelate can oblige his subject nor a father his son. The reason is both because the sick individual is not held to conserve the life of his body with such great pain and torture and because superiors cannot prescribe all things licit and honest but those only which are moderate.[23]

---

[22] "Non enim vitae conservandae gratia omnia media adhibenda sunt, sed illa tantum, quae ad hoc sunt necessaria et congrua." Ibid.

[23] "Ac proinde cum unisquissue jure naturali media licita, quae commode sumi possunt ad sui corporis conservationem ponere tenetur, peccaret sine dubio, qui absque magno dolore, cum possit saluti corporis succurrerer, se mori permitteret. Ad hoc tamen, ut ingentissimum dolorum in membri amputatione, vel corporis incisione ferret nec subditum praelatus, nec pater filium, obligare potest. Ratio est tum quia nec infirmus tenetur cum tanto dolore et cruciatu vitam corporis conservare. ...Tum

Before leaving the teachings of Sayrus, it is well to point
out that what was said earlier—regarding the fact that he in
many points merely repeats the writings of other authors—in
no way diminishes the value of his work. All through this
report the reader will see evidence of the effect that one writer
has had on another. To cite, however, the same doctrine as
each author comes into focus is not just simple repetition,
but rather an attempt to show the constant tradition that
has existed in this matter. Sayrus, for example, perhaps has
added very little original thought to this subject. His work
is of tremendous importance, nonetheless, because it mirrors
the opinions prevalent in his age regarding the necessity of
using the means of conserving one's life. Such will be the
case also as the different authors come up for review.

Among the commentators on the writings of St. Thomas,
one of the most famous is Domingo Bañez, O.P. (1528–1604).
Writing about St. Thomas's article on mutilation, Bañez treats
the question of whether or not the state can force a citizen to
undergo an amputation.[24] After this problem, he then places
the query before himself: "Is the man himself bound to suffer
the amputation of a member in order to save his life?"[25] In
response, he writes,

> It seems as though the answer is yes: because he is
> held to conserve his life through means which are
> ordered for this purpose and proportioned: but the
> cutting off of a member is a means proportioned to
> conserving life; therefore, he is bound to suffer the
> amputation. In answer here is the first conclusion.
> He is not bound absolutely speaking. The reason is

---

quia superiores non possunt omnia licita et honesta praecipere
sed ea tantum quae moderata sunt." Ibid., n. 38.

[24] Bañez, *Decisiones de iure et iustitia*, in II-II, q. 65, art. 1.

[25] "An ipsemet homo tenetur pati abscissionem membri
propter sevandam vitam?" Ibid.

that, although a man is held to conserve his own life, he is not bound to extraordinary means but to common food and clothing, to common medicines, to a certain common and ordinary pain: not, however, to a certain extraordinary and horrible pain, nor to expenses which are extraordinary in proportion to the status of this man. So that if, for example, it were certain that a common citizen would gain health if he spent three thousand ducats for a certain medicine, he would not be held to spend them. Thus, the argument is clear, for although that means is proportioned according to right reason and from the consequence is licit, it is, however, extraordinary.[26]

Tomás Sanchéz, S.J. (1550–1610), has substantially the same doctrine. This teaching is found in his famous *Consilia seu opuscula moralia*. Two of the more pertinent passages are the following:

One must suppose that it is one thing not to prolong life and it is another to shorten life. Let the first conclusion be: no one is held to prolong life,

---

[26] "Et videretur quod sic: quia tenetur servare vitam per media ordinata et proportionata: sed abscissio membri est medium proportionatum ad servandam vitam, ergo tenetur pati abscissionem. Repondetur et sit prima conclusio. Quod non tenetur absolute loquendo. Et ratio est quia quamvis homo teneatur conservare vitam propriam, non tenetur per media extraordinaria, sed per vitum et vestitum communem, per medicinas communes, per dolorem quendam communem et ordinarium: non tamen per quendam dolorem extraordinarium et horribilem, neque eitam per sumpus extraordinarios, secundum proportionem status ipsius hominis. Ut, si v.g., communem civem salutem consequuturum esset certum, si insumeret tria millia ducatorum in quadam medicina, illa non tenetur insumere. Per hoc patet ad argumentum, nam quamvis illud medium sit proportionatum secundum rectam rationem et ex consequenti licitum est tamen extraordinarium." Ibid.

indeed neither is he held to conserve it by using the best and most delicate foods; rather this is reprehensible. This is proved by reason of the fact that one is not bound to live in the most healthful place but can dwell in a region which is harmful due to the cold or heat; neither therefore is he held to seek out the most exquisite medicinal remedies, etc. Likewise, he is not bound to abstain from wine in order to live longer. . . . Hence the first inference that if one uses foods which men commonly use and in the quantity which customarily is sufficient for conserving strength, although he realizes due to this he will shorten his life considerably, he does not sin. Secondly, it is inferred that one is not obliged to use medicines to prolong life even where there would be the probable danger of death, such as taking a drug for many years to avoid fevers, etc. The second conclusion: one is held however, while sick, to consult doctors and use what is healthful.[27]

Further on he writes,

It is licit to fast and abstain even from common foods, not only in regard to the plurality of meals

---

[27] "Supponendum est aliud esse non prolongare vitam et aliud abbreviare vitam. Sit prima conclusion. Nullus tenetur prolongare vitam, immo nec illam conservare utendo optimus et delicatissimis alimentis, immo hoc est reprehensible. Probatur quia non tenetur abstinere a vino ut diutius vivat. . . . Hinc infertur primo, quod si quis utitur alimentis, quibus hominess communiter utunter et in quantine, quae solet sat esse ad valitudinem conservandam, licet pericipiat, ex hoc abbreviare vitam notabiliter, non peccat. Secundum infertur, quod non tenetur quis uti medicinis ad prolongandam vitam etiam ubi esset periculem probabile mortis, ut quotannis sumere pharmacum ad vitandas febres etc. Secunda conclusio, tenetur taman quis dum morbo laborat, consulere, medicos et uti cibis salutaribus." T. Sanchéz, *Consilia seu opuscula moralia* (Lyon, 1681), tom. II, lib. V, cap. 1, dub. 33, nn. 1–5.

but also in regard to the quantity, as long as the food necessary for the nourishment and conservation of the individual is taken. ... This is proved by reason of the fact that this is not to intend to abbreviate life or kill one's self but it is only to use means directed by nature for sustenance and not to prolong life, to which no one is bound, as I said.[28]

Francisco Suárez, S.J. (1548–1617), has a very interesting article which treats of the necessity that a man has of guarding his life. The question proposed is whether a man is bound to think of himself rather than his neighbor when a situation of danger to his own temporal goods arises.[29] Naturally, his life comes into question here. A good deal of the discussion would not be to the point just now, but there are a few passages which are of interest and which will prove helpful later:

The reason is that although a man may never kill himself, he is not bound, however, to conserve his life always and by every means, even by taking less account of the life of a neighbor, especially a friend or father.[30]

---

[28] "Licitum est jejunare et abstinere etiam a communibus cibus, non tantum, quo ad pluralitatem comestionum sed etiam quantum ad quantitatem, dummodo sumatur cibus necessarius ad alimentum et conservationem individiu. ... Probatur, quia hoc non est intendere abbreviare vitam, seu occidere se, sed tantum est uti mediis ordinatis a natura ad sustentationem et non prolongare vitam, ad quod nullus tenetur ut dixi." Ibid.

[29] F. Suarez, *Opera omnia*, ed. C. Berton (Paris, 1858), tom. XII, disp. 9, sect. 3.

[30] "Ratio est quia licet homo nunquam possit se occidere, non tamen semper, et omni medio, et ratione tenetur servare vitam, etiam postponendo vitam proximi, praecipue amici, vel patris." Ibid.

Again he writes,

> Without mortal sin, even in extreme necessity, one
> may take less account of himself in order to assist
> any other neighbor, even a stranger, in similar neces-
> sity. By the way of conclusion, it must be noted that
> we are speaking with only the consideration of char-
> ity in mind; for it is otherwise if the obligation of
> another virtue comes into question, as for instance
> justice or piety, as if he is the father of a family who
> is bound to make provisions and conserve himself
> for his sons and family."[31]

Another interesting sentence is, "Since mutilation in a prin-
cipal member is almost equivalent to death, for this reason a
man is not bound to undergo it in order to save his life."[32]

Straight away, one can recognize that a problem that
perplexed the moralists of this age was the doubt about
whether anyone could be forced to submit to an amputation
in order to save his life. Interesting speculation arose around
this problem, and in it, the writers have left indirectly, if not
directly, their teaching on the ordinary and extraordinary
means of conserving one's life. A good example of these is
Leonardus Lessius, S.J. (1554–1623):

> Notice that a man is bound to permit a member to
> be cut from him if the doctors judge this necessary
> and he will not have to suffer great pains. ... The

---

[31] "Potest quis sine peccato mortali in necessitate etiam
extrema se postponere, ut simili necessitate cujuvis alterius
proximi etiam extranei subveniat. Advertendum pro conclusione
est, nos loqui considerata propria sola ratione charitatis; nam
secus est si intercedat obligatio alterius virtutis, ut justitiae, vel
pietatis, ut si sit paterfamilias, qui ex officio tenetur providere,
et se conservare pro filiis et familia." Ibid., conclu. 4

[32] "Et quia multilatio in membro principali quasi aequipa-
ratur morti; unde non tenetur homo illam pati ut vitam servet."
Ibid., conclu. 5.

reason is that he is bound to help his endangered life by ordinary means which are not extremely difficult. If, however, tremendous tortures have to be suffered, he is not held to permit this nor can he be forced to this. The reason is because no one is obliged to conserve his life through such torture with an uncertain result.[33]

Lessius makes two exceptions, however. The first is the individual who is necessary for the common good. This person is bound to conserve his life even if an amputation is necessary, and it is the opinion of Lessius that he can be forced to submit to it by the State. The second exception involves the religious who is entirely under the power of his Superior. However, even Lessius doubts if this second exception is valid, because he does not feel that a Superior could licitly command under obedience so heroic an undertaking.[34]

When discussing the problem of impure touches and glances, Lessius brings up the question of whether or not a virgin, in order to conserve her life, is bound to undergo treatment from a male doctor in the more private parts of her body when such treatment would be a cause of intense embarrassment and shame. He replies,

Women, especially virgins, are not bound to accept from men medical treatment of this type in the more secret parts. ... The reason is because no one

---

[33] "Adverte hominem teneri permittere sibi membrum secari, si medici id judicent necessarium, nec magni dolores sint preferendi. ... Ratio est quia tenetur vitae suae periclitanti, emdiis ordinariis non admodum difficilibus opitulari. Si tamen ingentes essent cruciatus tolerandi, non tenetur permittere, neque etiam potest ad hoc cogi. Ratio est quia non tenetur quisquam cum tanto cruciatu vitam incerto eventu conservare." L. Lessius, *De justitia et jure* (Leuven, 1605), lib. II, cap. 9, dub. 14, n. 96.

[34] Ibid.

is held to accept a cure which he abhors no less than the disease itself or death: but many modest virgins prefer to tolerate a disease or death rather than to be touched by men. Furthermore, no one is obliged to accept that to which is conjoined the danger of an evil motion or carnal pleasure; indeed, it pertains to the heroic grade of chastity to prefer death rather than permit in one's self evil imaginations or any sense of evil desires.[35]

Martino Bonacina (d. 1631) also writes concerning the necessity of submitting to an amputation:

It is licit to amputate a member or a part of a member from one's self when such an amputation is necessary for the health of the whole body. Indeed, in such an event, there is an obligation of amputating if in the judgment of the doctor the pains are slight. The reason is that a man is bound to help his endangered life by ordinary remedies which are not too difficult; when, therefore, a certain member is injurious to the whole body, the law of nature dictates that it be cut off in order that we may help our life.[36]

---

[35] "Mulieres, praesertim virgins, non teneri huismodi genus medicandi in locis secretioribus a viris admittere. ... Ratio est, quia nemo tenetur admittere curationem, a qua non minus abhorret quam ab ipds morbo, vel morte: at multae virgines pudicae malunt tolerare morbum, vel mortem quam a viris contingi. Deinde nemo tenetur admittere id, cui conjunctum est periculum turpis motus, aut delectationis carnalis: imo ad heroicum castitatis gradum pertinet malle, mori quam permittere in se turpes imagines aut sensum ullum libidinis." Ibid., lib. IV, cap. 3, dub. 8, n. 60.

[36] "Licitum est sibi amputare membrum, vel membri partem, quando illius amputatio necessaria est ad salutem totius corporis. Imo, in tali eventu extat obligatio amputandi si dolores sint exigui, ita judicante medico. Ratio est quia homo tenetur vitae suae periclitanti opitulari remediis ordinariis non valde difficulibus, quando igitur membrum aliquod est toti corpori perniciosum jus naturae

Similarly, Paul Laymann, S.J. (1574–1635), writes,

> The second resolution is that we are not obliged for the most part to free our life from a disease or extrinsic violence by a means which is very difficult or not customary; e.g., by cutting off the feet or by using very precious medications. The reason is that the precept of preserving life is affirmative, not obliging in all times and in every way.[37]

In the *De justitia et jure* of Gabrielis a S. Vincentio, O.C.D. (d. 1671), the same doctrine is found:

> In the seventh place, you ask whether one is obliged to yield to a doctor or surgeon who judges that it is necessary for the conservation of the whole life that a leg or arm or other member be amputated? The response is affirmative when this can happen without great pain; the reason is that no one is held to take care of his life by extremely troublesome means nor by extremely torturous ones as neither by extremely costly means. Hence, I said that a certain nun was not obliged to reveal to a surgeon a disease which she had in the more secret parts of her body, because of the excessive modesty ("verecundia") which appeared to her to be more serious than death itself.[38]

---

dictat abscindendum esse, ut bitae opitulemus." M. Bonacina, *Moralis theologica* (Lyon, 1645), tom. Ii, disp. 2, quaest. ultim., sec. 1, punct. 6, n. 2.

[37] "Resolvitur secundo: Quod propriam vitam a morbo vel extrinseca violentia plerumque liberare non tenemur per medium valde difficile et insolitum; v.g. pedum sectione, medicamentis pretiosissimis. Ratio est: quod praeceptum servandi vitam affirmativum sit, non omni tempore ac modo obligans." P. Laymann, *Theologica moralis* (Munich, 1626), lib. III, tract. 3, p. 3, cap. 1, n. 4.

[38] "Quaeres 7 an teneatur quis parere medico, vel chirurgo judicanti necessarium esse pro totius vitae conservarione, quod

Late Seventeenth to
Nineteenth Centuries

The first section of Cardinal de Lugo's tenth disputation in his *De iustitia et iure* (1642) has for its title "Whether it is licit for a man to kill or mutilate himself."[39] Throughout this section de Lugo treats the many problems that concern suicide, mutilation, and the conservation of one's life. In the first chapter we have made mention of de Lugo's approach to the question of suicide. Here what is of interest is his treatment of the obligation that an individual has to conserve his own life and the necessity of using the means thereto. In the course of this section, de Lugo discusses a good number of particular cases. His solutions enable one to gather his teaching on the obligation of using the ordinary means of conserving life and the lawfulness of not employing the extraordinary means.

In no. 21, de Lugo reviews the malice of mutilation. Just as a man does not possess full dominion over his life, so also he lacks complete power over his members. Therefore, any mutilation that is not justified by the necessity of his body's health is illicit. Here, too, he explains what he understands by mutilation: to take away a member from one's self.[40] Since the necessity of mutilation for the conservation

---

crus, vel brachium, aut aliud membrum amputetur? Resp. affirmative, quando id fieri potest sine magne dolore, ratio est, quia nullus tenetur tueri vitam per media valde laboriosa, nec valde cruciativa, sicut neque per media ulde pretiosa. Hinc dixi non fuisse obliagatam quandam monilemostendere chirurgo quendam morbum, quem habebat in partibus secretioribus ratione maximae verecundiae quae sibi gravior apparebat quam esset moris ipsa." Gabrielis a S. Vincentio, *De justitia et jure* (Rome, 1663), disp. 6, *De restitutione*, q. 6, n. 86.

[39] "Utrum liceat homini seipsum interficere, vel multilare." De Lugo, *De iustitia a iure*, disp. X.

[40] "Membrum aliquod sibi auferre." Ibid., n. 21.

of life can render the mutilation licit, is it ever obligatory to suffer it? (Here again is evidence of the traditional approach. First an author will treat of suicide and the necessity of self-conservation. Then almost automatically, the next question is mutilation and the conditions which make it not only licit but obligatory.) De Lugo answers that an individual is obliged to permit a mutilation as a means of cure when the doctors judge this necessary and when it can be performed without intense pain. If, on the other hand, the mutilation is accompanied by very intense pain, then of course it ceases to be obligatory, because it becomes an extraordinary means of conserving life:

> He must permit this cure when the doctors judge it necessary and when it can happen without intense pain, not if it is accompanied by very bitter pain; because a man is not bound to employ extraordinary and difficult means to conserve his life.[41]

Therefore, de Lugo exempts an individual from employing the extraordinary means of conserving his life. However, it could happen that some individual because of certain circumstances would be bound to employ the extraordinary means. For instance, in de Lugo's own words, this would apply to one "whose life is very necessary for the public good."[42]

It has been seen even thus far that a discussion of mutilation among the authors of this age usually included some speculation on whether a religious, or for that matter, any person could be forced by the proper authority to submit to a mutilation in order to conserve his life. De Lugo mentions it too. He mentions the religious who is bound by a vow to

---

[41] "Debere eam curationem permittere, quando medici necessarium judicarent, et absque intenso dolore fieri posset; secus si acerbissimo dolore fieret; quia non tenetur homo media extraordinaria et difficillima adhibere ad vitae conservationem." Ibid.

[42] "Cuius vita bono publico sit valde necessaria." Ibid.

obey his Superior. Now, supposing that an amputation of some limb is necessary for the health of that religious, and his Superior orders him to undergo it. Must he do so? De Lugo cites the fact that some hold that the religious is bound to submit, even in this case, to the will of his Superior. However, he judges that the opposite opinion is more probable:

> Some accept also that the religious is obliged to obey his Superior who commands that he undergo the necessary amputation of a limb. Others, and more probably, deny this because such difficult things seem beyond the items of the rule in which religious are bound to obey.[43]

Then de Lugo interjects a thought of great importance. He states that this religious would be held to undergo the amputation, however, if he were necessary to the State or the Community and, he adds, "the remedy were entirely secure and certain."[44] Notice that this last element was mentioned also by Lessius when he taught that "no one is obliged to conserve his life under such torture with an uncertain result."[45] Even Vitoria, much earlier, had insinuated the same when he demanded that there be a hope of life, which rightly interpreted would seem to mean a hope of recovery.[46]

---

[43] "Aliqui excipiunt etiam religiosum, qui obedire debet praelato praecipienti, quod eismodi membri sectionem necessariam sustineat. Alii probabilius id negant, quia res adeo difficiles videntur esse extra res contentas in regula, in quibus religiosi obedire tenentur." Ibid.

[44] "Nisi religiosus necessarius esset reipublicae, vel communitati, et remedium esset omnino securum et certum." Ibid.

[45] "Non tenetur quisquam cum tanto cruciatu vitam incerto eventu conservare." Lessius, *De justitia et jure*, lib. II, cap. 9, cub. 14, n. 96.

[46] "Si aegrotus potest sumere cibum vel alimentum cum aliqua spe vitae, tenetur summere cibum." Vitoria, *De temperantia*, n. 1.

In succeeding numbers, de Lugo treats different problems regarding the unlawfulness of certain types of mutilation and suicide.[47] Not all of this is to the point here. However, in no. 28 he outlines the distinction between the positive and negative influences that an individual can have on his own death.[48] There are two ways in which a man sins against the obligation of conserving his life. The first is in a positive way, by performing something that will bring on death. The second is in a negative manner, that is, by not fleeing the danger of death when this can be accomplished easily:

> Note that a man sins against the obligation of conserving his life, first in a positive way, by doing something that is inductive of death, as for example, to pierce one's self with a sword, to cast one's self into a fire or a river, etc. Secondly, in a negative manner, by not fleeing the dangers of death, as when seeing a raging lion coming to devour him, an individual wills to wait unmoved although he could turn away and flee; or when seeing a fire already approaching him, he does not will to move from his place but awaits the flames.[49]

De Lugo admits that in this latter situation a man cannot be said to bring about his death in a positive manner,

---

[47] De Lugo, *De justitia et jure*, nn. 22–27.

[48] Ibid., n. 28, which has this title in the edition cited: "Alius est concursus positivus ad propriam mortem, alius negativus."

[49] "Adverte, dupliciter posse hominem pecare contra obligationem conservandi vitam, primo positive aliquid faciendo inductivum mortis, ut si ferro se percutiat, si in ignem se conjiciat vel in flumen, etc. Secundo negative, hoc est, non figiendo pericula mortis, ut si videns leonem furiosum ad ipsum devorandum venire, et potens facile decinare et fugere, velit immobilis expectare: vel si videns incendium jam ad ipsum appropinquare, nolit loci moveri, sed flammam expectare." Ibid., n. 28.

that is, by exerting some positive influence himself. Nonetheless, because the individual does not flee the cause of death when this is possible "in an ordinary and easy way,"[50] his behavior is "against the common obligation of caring for one's own life."[51]

In which category should the individual be placed who abstains from food necessary to sustain his life? De Lugo answers that "to abstain from food necessary for the sustenance of life when a person can sustain his life by ordinary means would pertain to the first genus."[52] Hence, for de Lugo, the refusal to employ the ordinary means (in this case, food) when this can be accomplished easily and in a normal manner is equivalent to performing an act which has a positive influence in bringing about one's own death.

Another important distinction is next outlined by de Lugo. He points out that danger of death can come from two different types of causes. The first is a natural and purely necessary cause, such as a flood or a fire. Danger of death arising from such a cause, one must attempt to escape. It would not be lawful to await its eventual destructive force. The second is a free cause, such as when one knows that an individual is intent on killing one. In this case the person concerned would not always be bound to flee but for a proportionately grave reason could await possible death. In other words, the obligation of fleeing the danger is greater in the first instance:

---

[50] "Ipsum tamen non fugere et declinare modo ordinario et facili mortem advenientem." Ibid.

[51] "Est contra obligationem communem tuendi propriam vitam." Ibid.

[52] "Ad hoc autem primum genus pertineret abstinere a cibo necessario ad vitam sustentandam quando facile potest mediis ordinariis illam sustentare." Ibid.

Again it seems that a distinction has to be made concerning this obligation of conserving life. For sometimes the danger comes from natural and purely necessary causes, sometimes from free causes. In the first case the obligation is greater: e.g., if a flood from a river or sea, or a fire approaches you, you cannot await it but you must flee lest it encompass you. . . . In the second case, however, there is not so great an obligation: e.g., if you know that someone is seeking to kill you . . . you are not held always to flee, but for a grave reason you can patiently await the death inflicted or to be inflicted by another.[53]

De Lugo offers a reason for his reply. In the first case, the natural and necessary cause is determined in itself and does not operate with any indifference. Therefore, the one who wills the necessary cause would seem to will its effect also. Such being the case, a man could really be called the author of his own death, since he wills the set of causes from which death necessarily arises. Certainly he does not will to impede it when he easily could. The second case is different because there is a question of a free cause. Since an effect follows a free cause contingently and not of necessity, it is not necessarily true that a person who would not flee such a cause would will its effect. Rather, he only permits this effect, if it should occur. In such a case, he would not be the author of his own death:

---

[53] " Rursus circa hanc obligationem conservandi vitam distinguendum videtur. Aliquando enim periculum provenit ex causis naturalibus et mere nessessariis: aliquando vero ex causis liberis. In primo casu obligatio est major: si v.g. inundatio fluminis vel maris, aut incendium ad te appropinquat, non potes illud expectare, sed debes fugere ne te comprehendat . . . in secundo autem casu non est tanta obligatio v.g. si scis aliquem te ad necam quaerere . . . non teneris semper fugere, sed potes ex causa gravi patienter mortem ab alio illatam vel inferendam expectare." Ibid., n. 29.

The point of difference in the two cases seems to be that in the first case, he who wills the necessary cause seems to will the effect, since a natural and necessary cause is determined in itself and does not operate with indifference: therefore, a man seems to be the author of his death when he wills the complexity of causes from which death arises, or certainly he does not will to impede it when he easily could. In the second case, however, since a free cause intervenes from which an effect follows contingently, it is not necessary that he will the effect when he does not flee this cause, but he holds himself permissive in relation to it. ... Hence, the man is not the author of his death.[54]

The point of main concern in the foregoing discussion is the emphasis which de Lugo places on the necessity of conserving one's life. It will also prove helpful later to have the clear distinction between natural and free causes in mind. So often in the disputations in theology, confusion arises because of the lack of clear-cut distinctions. This is true also in the matter of ordinary and extraordinary means.

For de Lugo then, the necessity of conserving one's life by ordinary means is beyond dispute. Not to use the ordinary means is the same as to inflict death on one's self:

I said, however, that a man must guard his life by ordinary means against dangers and death coming

---

[54] Ratio differentia inter utrumque casum haec videtur esse, quod in primo casu, qui vult causam necessarium, videtur velle effectum ipsum, cum causa naturalis et necessaria determinata sit ex se, et non operetur cum indifferentia: quare tunc homo videtur auctor esse suae mortis, cum velit eam complexionem causarum, exqua necessario mors oritur, vel certe non vult illam impedire, cum facile possit. In secundo autem casu, cum interveniat causa libera, ex qua contingenter sequitur effectur, non est necesse quod velit affectum qui non fugit illam causam, sed solum permissive se habet respectu illius. ... Unde homo tunc non est auctor suae mortis." Ibid.

from natural causes . . . because the one who neglects the ordinary means seems to neglect his life and therefore to act negligently in the administration of it, and he who does not employ the ordinary means which nature has provided for the ordinary conservation of life is considered morally to will his death.[55]

Such is not the case, however, with the extraordinary means of conserving life. In this paragraph, de Lugo gives a minor discussion on the nature of extraordinary means and the reason why they are not obligatory. However brief the discussion, his teaching is of great importance and assistance to one trying to determine the nature of the extraordinary means of conserving life. First of all, de Lugo rules out the necessity of any extraordinary diligence in accomplishing the conservation of life. For him, there is a clear distinction between the blameworthy neglect of one's life and the necessary care of it by very extraordinary means. The reason which de Lugo gives is that the "bonum" of a man's life is not so tremendously important that it demands conservation by all possible means. Perhaps this statement may appear a bit shocking at first. Rightly interpreted, however, its meaning is clear.

The affirmative precept of the natural law obliging conservation of one's life does not bind in the presence of a proportionately grave difficulty. Not every possible means must be employed, but only those which ordinary diligence requires. If in using ordinary means death occurs, his death

---

[55] "Dixi tamen, contra pericula, et mortem ex causis naturalibus provenientem debere hominem *mediis ordinaries,* vitam tueri ... quia qui media ordinaria negligit, videtur negligere vitam, atque ideo negligentem se in ejus gubernatione gerere, et moraliter censetur velle mortem, qui mediis ordinariis non utitur, non utitur, quae natura providit ad ordinariam vitae conservationem." Ibid.

nevertheless cannot be imputed to the individual as morally culpable:

> He is not held to the extraordinary and difficult means ... the "bonum" of his life is not of such great moment, however, that its conservation must be effected with extraordinary diligence: it is one thing not to neglect and rashly throw it away, to which a man is bound: it is another however, to seek after it and retain it by exquisite means as it is escaping away from him, to which he is not held; neither is he on that account considered morally to will or seek his death.[56]

De Lugo applies the principle again and says that in a situation where life is being taken away by another man, "you are not held to the ordinary means of fleeing death, except *per accidens* in a particular case on account of the inconveniences which will follow from your death."[57] The reason is that as far as the individual is concerned, he is conserving his life and the responsibility for death lies with the other person.[58]

A teaching of momentous importance is found under no. 30 in de Lugo's treatment of ordinary and extraordinary means. He supposes a situation in which a person is con-

---

[56] "Nec etiam tenetur ad media extraordinaria et difficilia ... non tamen est tanti momenti hoc vitae bonum ut extraodinaria diligentia procuranda sit ejus conservatio: aliud est eam non negligere et temere projicere, ad quod homo tenetur: aliud vero est eam quaerer et fugientem ex se retinere mediis exquisitis, ad quod non tenetur, nec ideo censetur moraliter mortem velle aut quarerere." Ibid.

[57] "Nec ad ordinaria media teneris ut mortem fugias, nisi per accidens in aliquo casu propter inconvenientia quae ex tua morte sequuntur." Ibid.

[58] "Quia tunc jam quantam ex te est, vitam conservas, nec ex te provenit ejus amissio, sed ex alio quod tibi non imputatur, sed illi." Ibid.

demned to death by fire. While surrounded by the flames, he notices that he has sufficient water to extinguish some of the fire but not all of it. Must he use this water? De Lugo says no, and gives his reason:

> If a man condemned to fire, while he is surrounded by the flames, were to have at hand water with which he could extinguish the fire and prolong his life, while at the same time other wood is being carried forward and burned, he would not be held to use this means to conserve his life for such a brief time because the obligation of conserving life by ordinary means is not an obligation of using means for such a brief conservation—which is morally considered nothing at all.[59]

However, if he could put the fire out once and for all, and thus escape death, it would seem that the use of the water would be obligatory, because then his death could not be considered as coming absolutely from an extrinsic source "since there would be left to him the free ability of defending himself from the fire by ordinary means."[60] In other words, here again the element of benefit is introduced. The means and remedies employed, even though in themselves common and ordinary, must offer some hope of benefit or help to the conservation of life before they become obligatory. Furthermore, this benefit must be of some considerable duration—in other words, proportionate.

---

[59] "Si enim quis ad ignem damnatus, dum jam flamma circumdatus est haberet ad manum aquam, qua posset ignem extinguere et vitam protrahere, quamdiu alia ligna afferuntur et accenduntur; non ideo teneretur ei medio uti, ut vitam illo brevi tempore conservaret: quia obligatio utendi mediis ad illam brevem conservationem quae moraliter pro nihilo reputatur." Ibid., n. 30.

[60] "Cum relinqueretur ei facultas libera defendendi se ab igne media ordinaria." Ibid.

Otherwise, if the profit from using these means is only brief, then for de Lugo it must be considered of no value morally and thus not obligatory. "Parum pro nihio reputatur."

De Lugo also treats the opinion already reviewed here that a man is not bound to effect a prolongation of his life by using choice and delicate foods. In similar fashion, neither is he bound to abstain from wine in order to live longer. He expresses it as follows:

> Whence, much less is a man bound to effect a lengthening of his life by choice and delicate foods, for just as one is not held to abstain from wine in order to live longer, so neither is he bound to drink wine for the same purpose: because just as a man is not bound to seek a more healthful and wholesome locality and air in order to prolong his life, so neither is he held to eat better or more healthful food.[61]

The reader has, without doubt, taken note that the theologians cited thus far, when discussing ordinary means, have constantly referred to a comparison with the manner in which men commonly live.[62] An interesting application of this principle occurs in de Lugo. He repeats the difference between bringing about one's own death in a positive manner and omitting the use of certain means of conserving life. The first is never licit; the second can be licit in certain

---

[61] "Unde multo minus tenetur homo vitae elongationem procurare cibis exquisitis et delicatis, sicut enim non tenetur quis abstinere a vino, ut longius vivat, sic nec vinum libere ad eundem finem: quia sicut non tenetur homo salubriorem locum, et aerem quaerere ad vitam prolongandam, sic nec meliorem et salubriorem victum sumere." Ibid., n. 32.

[62] "Juxta communem doctorum sentintiam, non est obligatio utendi medicina exquisita et pretiosa ad vitandum mortem." Ibid., n. 36.

circumstances. In harmony with this principle, therefore, according to the common opinion of the doctors, there is no obligation of using choice and costly medicine to avoid death. This omission does not imply a direct killing of one's self, but rather the person concerned permits his death and rests content with using only the ordinary and common means by which men commonly live.[63] Hence, the person does not positively influence his death but dies on account of old-age or the weakness of his own life.[64] With this in mind therefore, we may conclude that a religious novice would not be bound to return to the world to eat better and seek other conveniences for the sake of his health when those in religion do not commonly live in that manner.[65] Here is the interesting application made by de Lugo, because he is obviously taking the measure of comparison from the surroundings which are required by the individual's state in life. Hence, although strictly speaking, given that the common food for common men living in the world may be an ordinary means for them, it nevertheless remains extraordinary for the religious who in his cloister would not ordinarily eat in the manner ordinary or customary in the world.

The foregoing report on the teaching of de Lugo reveals his strict adherence to the traditional doctrine in these matters. Likewise, it shows the clever and precise explanations

---

[63] "Haec enim omittere non est se occidere, sed permittere mortem ex se obvenientem, et relinquere se ordinariis et communibus mediis, quibus alii homines communiter vivunt." Ibid.

[64] "Neque enim hic se occidit, sed moritur propter aegritudinem, vel infirmitatem suae maturae." Ibid.

[65] "Cur ergo novitus tenebitur sub peccato dire in saeculum, ut quaerat delicias, delicatos cibos, et luxem, nec satisfaciet utendo victu, et mediis quibus alii communiter in religione utuntur et vitam conservant?" Ibid.

and applications of the principles involved which de Lugo makes, all of which will be of assistance further on in this dissertation.

It is the same doctrine that is given by Anthony Diana (1585–1663). Citing Vitoria, he admits that a sick person for whose health there is no hope can refuse to buy a costly drug that will prolong his life for some days, even though he is able to buy it.[66] Diana also follows previous teaching in the matter of mutilation. Even though an amputation is necessary for the health of the individual, he need not feel obliged to suffer it when it is accompanied by intense pain and torture.[67] Actually, Diana is more forthright than his predecessors when he includes in this exception the religious bound by obedience. He says categorically that the religious is not bound to the amputation and cannot be forced to it, "even if … the Superior commands this [surgery] to him."[68]

Each theologian makes a contribution in his writings. Many in the matter of the ordinary and extraordinary means of conserving life have perhaps served only to reflect the teachings prevalent in their age. Others carry on the existing tradition and add a different approach or solve a different case. Some perhaps even point out a new problem. Others relate the old teaching in a more precise manner.

---

[66] "Et idem Vitoria ait, licet aegrotus, di cuius salute desperature, posset aliquot dies pharmaco protrahere vitam, non teneri illud emere." A. Diana, *Coordinatus*, ed. Martin de Alcolea (Lyon, 1667), tom. VIII, tract. V, res. 53 (ex Diana, p. 5, tr. 4, res. 33).

[67] "Hominem teneri permittere sibi membrum secari, si medici id judicent necessarium, nec magni dolores sint perferendi, si tamen ingentes essent cruciatus tolerandi … non tenetur permittere, neque potest ad hoc cogi." Ibid., res. 57.

[68] "Etiam si Religiosus et Superior id ei praeciperet." Ibid.

Honoré Tourney (1658–1729) in his *Theologica moralis* reiterates much of what went before him. For instance, he excludes the necessity of using very costly medications which would consume a considerable amount of one's resources. Neither is it obligatory to undergo very intense pain such as in the amputation of feet or arms.[69] Tourney not only excludes the necessity of using these means but also assigns the reason: "Means of this type are morally impossible."[70]

Interestingly enough, this author next discusses the person who does not agree to suffer even moderate pain in order to conserve his life. Can he be forced to submit to an amputation if it involves only moderate pain? Tourney's answer is that this individual can be forced by those who are entrusted with his care, or even by someone acting in virtue of a mandate from such persons. Tourney is hesitant about enlarging the circle of those who have the authority to command such a procedure.[71] However, what is of importance is the fact that Tourney recognizes and teaches that moderate pain does not constitute moral impossibility and hence, generally speaking, does not make a means extraordinary.

The Carmelite Fathers of Salamanca, known as the Salmanticenses, have this precise wording of the doctrine on the ordinary and extraordinary means of conserving life:

---

[69] "Sic non habetur ut homicida sui, qui abstinet a pretiosissimis medicamentis, in quibus profundi deberent opes patrimonii; item qui non vult gravissimos cruciatus pedum v.g. vel brachiorum sectionem patri, ut vitam diutius protrahat." H. Tourney, *Theologica moralis* (Venice, 1756), tom. III, tract. de decalogo, cap. 2, de quinto praec., art. I, conc. 2.

[70] "Cum huiusmodi media moraliter impossibilia sint." Ibid.

[71] "Sed quid si homo ne moderatos quidem dolores pati velit, ut vitam servet, poteritne invitus abscindi? Poterit ad iis aut de mandato eorum, qui curam ejus gerunt, ut pater, tutor, Superior, et similes: an autem et ab aliis mutilari possit, non ita constat." Ibid.

Also, in order to conserve his life, one is not bound to use all possible remedies, even extraordinary ones, really choice medicines, costly foods, a transfer to more healthful territory, so that he will live longer: he is not held to give over all his wealth in order to avoid death which is threatened by another person, whether justly or unjustly: neither is a sick individual in desperate condition bound to employ very costly remedies, even though he should know that with these remedies his life would be extended for some hours or days or even years.[72]

The intense pains of amputation excuse a person from the obligation of employing such a remedy for the further conservation of his life. In this the Salmanticenses adhere to previous teachings. Likewise, they make only one exception, and state that a person who is necessary for the common good should submit to such a procedure in order to save his life. Furthermore, the proper authority can command him to submit.[73] However, they add, "if the remedy is entirely certain for the conservation of his life."[74] No one ordinarily, then, is bound to permit an amputation, "because—as the

---

[72] "Nec etiam tenetur aliquis ad conservandum vitam ut omnibus possibilibus remediis, etiam extraordinariis, nimirum exquisitis medicinis, cibis pretiosis, ire ad terras salubriores ad amplius vivendum: nec dare omnes suas divitias pro evitanda morte juste vel injuste ab alio minata: nec tenetur infrimus desperatus uti remediis pretiosissimis, tametsi cum illis sciret vitam per aliquas horas, vel dies, vel etiam annos fore extendendam." Salmanticenses, *Cursus theologiae moralis* (Lyon, 1879), tom. III, tract. XIII, de restit., cap. II, punct. 2, sect. 2, n. 26.

[73] "Nec tenetur infirmus eam patio ob conservationem vitae nec posset hoc Respublica, aut Praelatus illis praecipere, nisi esset persona multum neccessaria bono communi." Ibid., punct. 3, n. 50.

[74] "Si remedium esset omnino certum ad illius vitae conservationem." Ibid.

Roman said, the opening up of whose leg caused him intense pain, health is not worth such pain—no one is held to conserve his life by extraordinary and horrible means."[75]

The doctrine on the ordinary and extraordinary means of conserving life as found in the *Medulla theologiae moralis* of Hermann Busenbaum, S.J. (1600–1668), is merely a collection of all that has been reported here so far. It is known that the first edition of the *Moral Theology* of St. Alphonsus in 1748 actually was the *Medulla theologiae moralis* of Busenbaum, to which Alphonsus added certain notes.[76] Even in succeeding editions, Busenbaum's *Medulla* was the basis for Alphonsus's noted work. Especially in the matter of the ordinary and extraordinary means of conserving life, this is true. Hence it seems well to treat the writings of both these authors together.

In point of fact, nothing new is added by either of these authors in this matter. However, for future reference, it will be profitable here to outline the elements and conditions which these authors feel render a means of conserving life extraordinary. First of all, there is no obligation of using any costly and uncommon medicine.[77] There is no need of chang-

---

[75] "Quia, ut dicebat ille Romanus, cui crus cum ingenti dolore aperiebatur; 'non est tanto dolore digna salus'—non enim quis tenetur per media extraordinaria, et horrenda vitam conservare." Ibid.

[76] See Alphonsus, *Theologia moralis*, praefatio editoris, for a historical study of the editions of St. Alphonsus's *Theologia moralis* and the influence that the *Medulla* of Busenbaum exerted on St. Alphonsus.

[77] "Ideoque non teneri … nec aliquem alium uti pretiosa et exquisita medicina ad mortem vitandam." H. Busenbaum, *Medulla theologiae moralis* (Rome, 1757), lib. III., tract. IV, de quinto-sexto praecepto, cap. 1, n. 371; Alphonsus, *Theologia moralis*, lib. III, tract. IV, cap. 1, n. 371.

ing one's place of residence in order to get a more healthful climate outside one's native land.[78] No one is held to employ extraordinary and very difficult means, such as the amputation of a leg, in order to conserve his life.[79] True, the obligation of taking an expensive medicine does not exist, but if it is an ordinary medication one would be bound to employ this means of conserving his life provided that some hope of future health could be foreseen.[80] The abhorrence that a sick woman, particularly a maiden, might have for medical treatment by a male doctor or surgeon would seem to be sufficient, ordinarily speaking, to excuse her from this treatment.[81] However, if the services of a woman doctor or surgeon were available, certainly this treatment would be obligatory.[82]

As can be seen, both Busenbaum and Alphonsus adhered strictly to the traditional teaching on this subject. No doubt, it has become obvious to the reader by now that the moralists at this period are merely repeating the very same phrases and examples which their predecessors used. Perhaps the reason is that at this time there were other, more important problems confronting the moral theologians. Perhaps also progress in the medical field had not actually reached

---

[78] "Nec secularem, relicto domicilio, quaerere salubriorem aerem extra patriam." Busenbaum, n. 371; Alphonsus, n. 371.

[79] "Non teneri quemquam mediis extraordinariis, et nimis duris, v. gr. abscissione cruces, etc. vitam conservare." Busenbaum, n. 372, and Aphonsus, n. 372.

[80] "Infirmum in periculo mortis, si sit spes salutis non posse medicamina respuere." Ibid.

[81] "Non videtur tamen virgo aegrotans (per se loqundo) teneri subire manus medici vel chirurgic quando id ei qravissimum est, et magis quam mortem ipsam horret." Ibid.

[82] "Posset tamen virgo permittere tangi; immo teneretur sinere, ut ab alia femina curetur." Alphonsus, n. 372.

such a degree as to initiate any speculation on whether a particular remedy should be considered obligatory or not. Evidently an amputation during this period in history was the perfect example of a terrible torture which no one ordinarily could be held to undergo. When, evidently, an interpretation of the obligations imposed by religious obedience presented a problem in this matter, the theologians solved it. Had doctors and other scientists created doubts or difficulties by advancing new and secure methods of heath and cure, no doubt these very moralists would have settled them, as they did in so many other instances. The absence of speculation therefore seems due to the fact that difficulties in the matter were not presented to the moralists, rather than to any want of appreciation of the problem itself.

Antonio de Escobar, S.J. (1589–1669), took from Vitoria much of his teaching on the necessity of using the ordinary means of conserving life. He uses Vitoria's example of the man who, according to the judgment of a doctor, would be able to prolong his life ten years if he would drink wine. Escobar with Vitoria answers that this individual "can nevertheless abstain from the wine."[83]

This very same doctrine is taught by Tommaso Tamburini, S.J. (1591–1675), in his *Explicatio decalogi*.[84] This author also lists great pain as a cause excusing a man from undergoing an amputation, because charity in regard to your

---

[83] "Posse nihilominus a vino abstinere." A. de Escobar, *Universae theologiae moralis, receptiores absque lite sententiae nec non controversae disquisitiones* (Lyon, 1663), IV, lib. 32, cap. V, prob. XXIV, n. 128.

[84] "Qui te non obligat ad utendum vino, vel carnibus; etiamsi Medicas dicat te victurum cum illis amplius decem annis quam si utaris aqua et piscabus." T. Tamburini, *Explicatio decalogi* (Venice, 1719), lib. VI, cap. II, sect. II, n. 11.

own life is not demanded with such great inconveniences.[85] For that very reason, medication that can be obtained only at a high price is not obligatory.[86] Interestingly enough, Tamburini is quite realistic in his treatment of the necessity of undergoing an amputation. As has just been said, he teaches that it is not obligatory, but he takes note of the fact that many previous authors have excepted the individual who is necessary for the common good. Then Tamburini adds that this, "at least practically, does not apply because ordinarily you can prudently consider that when you die, another just as capable will take your place."[87]

The necessity of suffering a surgical intervention in order to conserve one's life is also excluded by Apollonius Holzmann, O.F.M. (1681–1749). For this author also, the obligation of conserving one's life does not require the use of extraordinary and very difficult means. Since a surgical section would involve pain and be in fact extraordinary, it cannot be said to be obligatory.[88] Patritius Sporer (d. 1683) in his *Theologia moralis* has the following very concise treatment. It is worthy of quotation, since he gives in this excerpt most of

---

[85] "Cum tanto incommodo non urget caritas in tuam ipsammet vitam." Ibid., sect. III, n. 3.

[86] "Nam propter eandem rationem modo diximus, non obligari nos medicamentis mango pretio conquisitis et extraordinariis vitam annosque protrahere." Ibid.

[87] "Saltem practice non urget, quia regulariter potes prodenter existimare, tibi morienti alterum non minus aptum successurum." Ibid.

[88] "Ratio est quia nemo per se loquendo, tenetur suam vitam conservare per media extraordinaria et admodum difficulia; cum non sit tanto digna dolore salus, juxta commune adagium: sed sectio est medium extraordinarium et admodum difficile—ergo." A. Holzmann, *Theologia moralis* (Benevento, 1743), vol. I, pars II, tract. II, disp. V, cap. III, cas. II.

the conditions which the moralists of his time considered the identification marks of extraordinary means:

> It is for this reason that they sin mortally who have a gravely dangerous or deadly disease and are not willing to employ the ordinary and conveniently procurable remedies, and thus having neglected these remedies, permit their death when it can be very conveniently and reasonably impeded; for, since we are not the masters of our lives, but the guardians only, we are bound to conserve our life only by means which are ordinary and *per se* directed to the conservation of life; not, in like manner, by means which are extraordinary, unusual and very difficult either because of suffering, e.g., in the amputation of a member, arm or leg, or because of price, e.g., a medicine which is too expensive considering one's position. ... The reason is because the precept of conserving life is affirmative, and therefore does not bind pro semper but only at certain times and in a certain manner.[89]

Among the conditions which could render a means extraordinary, there are three that Johann Georg (Anacleto) Reiffenstuel, O.F.M. (1641–1703), seems to emphasize. He

---

[89] "Quando nimirum commode et rationabiliter impediri potest: qua ratione peccant mortaliter, qui in qravi periculoso aut lethali morbo nolunt adhibere remedia ordinaria, et commodo parabilia, iisque neglectis mortem permittunt; cim enim non simus domini sed custodies tantum vitae nostrae, tenemur vitam nostram conservare mediis ordinariis, et per se ordinatis ad vitam conservandam tantum; non item mediis extraodinariis insolitis, multumqe difficilibus, aut ob cruciatum, v.g. abscissione membri, brachii, vel tibiae aut ob pretium v.g. medicina nimium sumptuosa comparatione sui status. ... Ratio est quia praeceptum servandi vitam affirmativum est, ideoque non pro semper sed certo tantum tempore et modo obligat." P. Sporer, *Theologica moralis* (Venice, 1766), tom. I, tract. V, cap. III, sect. I, n. 13.

gives a very precise discussion of the matter in his *Theologia moralis*.[90] First of all, no one is obliged to conserve his life except by means which are ordinary, considering his position or status. Secondly, there must be a considerable hope of recovery from the illness by using these means. Thirdly, Reiffenstuel requires that the individual be able to employ the means without tremendous difficulty. All three of these conditions must be fulfilled simultaneously in the same individual, otherwise the means is an extraordinary means of conserving life. These three conditions are not listed numerically in Reiffenstuel, as they have been here. Rather, they have been gathered from the elements included in a difficulty which he presents and answers in the negative:

> No one is bound to conserve his life except by means which are ordinary in respect to his status. ... Do not say: if no one is bound to conserve his life except by ordinary means, then a sick man without being accused of indirectly killing himself can in good conscience refuse medicines when in danger of death, even though these medicines are not too costly and, furthermore, even though there would be a great hope of recovery if he took the medicines, which he could do without tremendous difficulty.[91]

Reiffenstuel, quite significantly, finds no trouble in stating that the sick individual in the circumstances just outlined

---

[90] A. Reiffenstuel, *Theologia moralis* (Modena, 1740), tract. IX, distinc. III, quaes II, n. 14.

[91] "Quia nemo tenetur suam vitam servae nisi mediis respectu sui status ordinariis ... non dicas: Si nemo tenetur suam vitam servare, nisi mediis ordinariis, tunc aeqrotus, quin dicatur se ipsum indirecte occidere, potest bona conscienta respuere medicinas in periculo mortis, quamvis illae medicinae non sint nimium pretiosae et caeteroquin foret magna spes reconvalescentiae, si easdem, quas asque ingenti difficultate posset, etiam summeret." Ibid.

must accept the medicines because they are ordinary means of conserving his life and therefore obligatory.[92]

In his treatment of this problem, Claude Lacroix, S.J. (1652–1714) repeats much of what was written by the moralists before him. This is especially true since this author is basing his work on that of Busenbaum. Lacroix acknowledges his debt to such authors as Vitoria, Lessius, de Lugo, Laymann, and others.[93] For example, he mentions costly and choice medicines and voluntary exile from one's native land as examples of means which are not of obligation. One of the conditions that this moralist also requires before any means can be termed ordinary is the hope of deriving some good from the use of a remedy.

In a sort of postscript to this whole discussion, Lacroix has some speculation on just how great the obligation of conserving or prolonging one's life can be said to be.[94] First of all, he indicates that the obligation of prolonging one's own life is not the same as the obligation of conserving it. The reason is that the prolongation of life implies a singular assiduity to which we are not held, whereas the non-abbreviation or the conservation of life implies only a common diligence to which we are obliged."[95]

Later, Lacroix cites a dispute regarding the necessity of undergoing a surgical section or the amputation of a leg

---

[92]"Respond. enim negando illatum et eiusdem suppositum, quasi nimurum medicinae respectu status infirmorum essent quid extraordinarium: etenium hae, praesertim non ninmis pretiosae … non sunt extraordinaria sed potius ordinaria remeida." Ibid.

[93]See C. Lacroix, *Theologia moralis* (Ravenna, 1761), vol. I, lib. III, pars I, tract. IV, cap. I, dub. I.

[94]Ibid., addenda.

[95]"Ratio est *vitam prolongare* importat singulare studium, ad quod non tenemur, e contra *non abbreviare et conservare* importat commune tantum stadium ad quod tenemur." Ibid., n. 3.

when one foresees that the neglect of such a procedure could result in one's death. As to the obligation entailed, he writes, "Some say yes because you are not the master of your life; others say no because no one is held to employ extraordinary and very difficult means to conserve his life."[96]

Finally, it is well to note that this moralist considers the notion of incertitude when determining a means as ordinary or extraordinary. Giving reference to Vitoria, Lacroix says a man is not held to conserve his life by medicines, because it is uncertain whether the effects of a medicine will be good or bad. Actually we do not know whether medicines will prolong one's life or shorten it.[97]

The teaching of Constantino Roncaglia (1677–1737) follows the general outline of that of his predecessors. Ordinary means are obligatory, and extraordinary means are not usually of obligation. An individual cannot be said to be negligent in caring for his life if he employs the ordinary means. This is true because one could never be called negligent in this mode of acting "if he uses all those means which ordinarily are in use in any project to be undertaken."[98] However, one would not be obliged to use means which are very costly or very painful or means which cause great shame.[99]

Roncaglia agrees with the moralists before him that an amputation of a diseased member of the body would not usually be obligatory if it involved tremendous suffering.

------

[96] "Aliqui affirmant quia non es dominus vitae tuae; alii negant quia nemo tenetur media extraordinaria et valde difficilia adhibere ad conservandam vitam." Ibid., n. 16.

[97] See ibid., n. 6.

[98] "Si utatur iis omnibus, quae ordinarie sunt in usu in aliqua it peragenda." C. Roncaglia, *Theologia moralis* (Lucca, 1730), vol. I, tract. XI, cap. I, q. III.

[99] "Non vero extraordinariis et valde pretoisis sicut etiam valde doloriferis, seu magnam afferentibus erubescentiam." Ibid.

However, his teaching is not quite so unconditional in this matter as that of earlier authors. Regularly, the moralists cite an amputation as an example of extraordinary means. Roncaglia agrees with this if unbearable pain accompanies the cutting away of a limb. Whenever, however, "from the amputation, future pains of notable proportion will not arise but only moderate pains, then one is bound to suffer the abscission; for everyone is held to conserve his life by ordinary means and it is an ordinary means to suffer something to conserve this same life."[100]

Naturally enough, Roncaglia excludes the necessity of undergoing tremendous torments in order to conserve one's life. It is significant, however, that he is willing to distinguish surgical procedures into the type involving extraordinary pain and difficulty and the type involving only moderate pain. All previous theologians have recognized the distinction in theory. The application of it to a surgical section or abscission, however, is noteworthy and important. Roncaglia also underlines the necessity of suffering a moderate difficulty for the conservation of one's life. This too is of considerable import. Pain of itself does not render a means extraordinary. It must be a pain that will involve intense torment in such a way as to constitute a certain impossibility or unproportionate difficulty. All this was recognized by previous moralists, but it certainly is stated more precisely in Roncaglia.

In discussing the question of whether a sick man is bound to take means to gain his health again, Nicholas Mazzotta, S.J. (1669–1737), gives certain elements that would render a means extraordinary and thus not obligatory. First of all, if there is no hope of recovery, a means need not be

---

[100] "Ex abscissione non sint futuri dolores ingentes, sed moderati, tunc tenetur mediis ordinariis vitam conservare et medium ordinarium est aliquid pati pro eadem vita conservanda." Ibid., q. IV.

employed. Secondly, great horror or torment or extraordinary expenditure of money would excuse an individual from employing these means. The reason is that duty requires only ordinary diligence and expense. The use of extraordinary means is considered to involve some sort of impossibility. This teaching is found in Mazzotta's *Theologia moralis*.[101]

The traditional doctrine is also taught by Benjamin Elbel, O.F.M. (1690–1756), in his work on moral theology.[102] Likewise, Charles-René Billuart, O.P. (1685–1757) states that "they are guilty who, while they are sick, refuse common remedies which will certainly or more probably be of benefit and not harmful, if from the lack of these death results."[103] On the other hand, remedies which are unusual, very difficult, or very expensive, considering the person's status, are not of obligation, because we are held to conserve

---

[101] "Hinc tenetur cibum vel medicamentum sumere etc. si inde affulgeat spes vitae. Caeterum, si non posit ea sumere sine magna consternatione, cruciatu etc. non peccat, quia tunc reputatur impossibilitas quaedam. Item nec peccat, qui, etiamsi possit, non facit expensas extraordinarias pro medicis, medicamentis, etc. etiamsi prudenter timeatur mors; quia sufficit adhibere expensas et diligentiam ordinariam." N. Mazzotta, *Theologia moralis* (Venice, 1760), tom. I, tract. II, disp. II, quaest. I, cap. I.

[102] See B. Elbel, *Theologia moralis per modum conferentiarum*, ed. I. Bierbaum (Paderborn, 1891–1892), II, nn. 25, 27, and particularly 28: "Etiamsi quilibet teneatur conservare vitam suam mediis ordinariis secundum dicta, nullus tamen (per se, nisi scilicet bonum publicum, charitas erga Deum aut proximum aliud suadeat) teneatur in hunc finem uti mediis nimis difficilibus vel medicamentis extraordinariis seu etiam nimis sumptuosis."

[103] "Rei sunt qui dum aegrotant recusant remedia communia, certo seu probabilius profutura et non nocitura, si cx earum defectu mors sequatur." C. Billuart, *Summa S. Thomae* (Paris, 1852), tom. VI, dissert. X, art. III, consect. n. 3.

our lives only by ordinary means. Furthermore, "God does not command that we be solicitous of a longer life."[104]

Vincenzo Patuzzi, O.P. (1700–1769), agrees in general with the teaching of his predecessors in the matter of the ordinary and extraordinary means of conserving life. He holds that a sick person would not be bound to employ the extraordinary means. As examples of extraordinary means, he gives the abscission of a member, choice and more costly medicines, a long journey or absence from one's native land undertaken for the sake of a better climate, and finally grave expense.[105] The reason assigned by Patuzzi is that most of the remedies involve a difficulty which is too burdensome and may even produce harm. Furthermore, their results are uncertain and very often useless.[106] Even if, however, one would have a morally certain hope that the recovery of health would eventuate from the use of these means, an individual would not have to use them, because the law of charity and the natural law do not demand that he employ such extraordinary, harsh, and violent remedies in order to conserve his life.[107] The question is impractical anyway, according to Patuzzi, because people usually sin by being

---

[104] "Neque jubet Deus ut de vita longiore ita simul solliciti." Ibid.

[105] "Non tenetur infirmus saluti suae providere extraordinariis remediis, puta abscissione membri, exquisitis et pretioribus medicinis, longa a patria peregrinatione et absentia ob aeris mutationem, vel gravioribus expensis." V. Patuzzi, *Ethica Christiana sive theologia moralis* (Bassani, 1770), tom. III, tract. V, pars V, cap. X, consect. sept.

[106] "Quia haec remedia plurimum incommodi et damni afferunt, graviora et incerta sunt ac plerumque inutilia." Ibid.

[107] "Non ergo legem naturae et caritatis violabit qui recto fine justaque de causa remediis extraordinariis, acerbioribus et violentis vitam conservare recusarent." Ibid.

too solicitous of conserving their lives rather than the other way around.[108]

There is one notable departure from tradition in the writings of Patuzzi, however. He holds a stricter view regarding the maiden's obligation to accept treatment from a surgeon even at the price of great embarrassment and shame. Actually, it is not surprising to find that in this matter, one of his views is stricter than that of other moralists, because Patuzzi has somewhat of a reputation for being rigorous in his opinions.[109] It will be well though, to quote the passage in question, because it reveals a different approach, which Patuzzi borrowed from Angelo Franzoja (d. 1760):[110]

> I agree, however, with Franzoja when he teaches well that it is not licit for a girl to refuse the healing hand of a surgeon and thus undergo death because her shame or foolishness deem it something most grave and even more painful than death, since this is not in itself troublesome, harsh, or difficult but arises only from the imprudent and inane idea of the patient which she ought to subject to the law of charity and the law of nature; especially since the doctor's hand is not an extraordinary remedy but a common one, in itself simple and easily procurable; furthermore, one which by the law of nature and charity should be employed when necessity demands it.[111]

---

[108] See ibid.

[109] Lehmkuhl says of him, "In re morali rigidus, S. Alphonsi adversarius erat, quem scriptis impugnativ." *Theologia moralis*, II, p. 838.

[110] Regarding Franzoja, Lehmkuhl writes, "Paravit editionem theolgiae Lacroix et Zaccariae *cum notis* in quibus rigidissimum se ostendit." Ibid., p. 831.

[111] "Assentior tamen Franzojae optime docenti, non licere puellae recusare medicam Chirurgi manum ac proinde mortem subire, quia eius sive verecundiae, sive imbecillitati id gravissimum

Nineteenth Century to the Present

After St. Alphonsus, in the nineteenth century, the characteristics of the treatments given this problem of the ordinary and extraordinary means of conserving life were fairly well standardized. Alphonsus had emerged as a recognized authority and leader in the field of moral theology. What he had learned from the previous theologians was now to be passed down by the authors who followed him. This is particularly true regarding the problem of the ordinary and extraordinary means of conserving life. Here and there different speculation is discovered, but for the most part, the authors are content to paraphrase Alphonsus.

For example, writing his moral theology according to the teaching of Alphonsus, Pietro Scavini (1790–1869) says,

> But one is not held to the extraordinary (means), namely, when the remedy is very hard or very repugnant to modesty, unless his life is entirely connected with the common good. Hence, one is not held to conserve his life by the amputation of a leg or another operation of the same genus which involves pains entirely too intense, since this is beyond human endurance. In this case, [in] the common estimation of men, he is thought only to permit his death for a just cause.[112]

---

et etiam ipsa morte acerbius videtur cum hoc non in se molestum, asperum, arduumque sit, sed ex sola patientis imprudenti et inani apprehensione oritur, quam legi caritatis et naturae subjicere debet; praesertim cum medica manus non extraordinarium remedium sit, sed commune & in se facile ac obvium; proinde necessitate urgente lege naturae et caritatis adhibendum." Patuzzi, *Ethica Christiana*, tom. III, tract. V, pars V, cap. X, consect. sept.

[112] "Sed non tenetur ad extraordinaria, nempe quoties remedium durissimum est; vel pudori valde repugnans: nisi ejus vita bono communi sit omnino conducens. Hinc non tenetur quis abscissione cruris, vel alia ejusdem generis operatione dolores

Another author of great importance is John Gury, S.J. (1801–1866). Gury mentions in his *Compendium theologiae moralis* that severe pain[113] would render a means extraordinary; as an example, he cites the amputation of a leg or arm or an incision into the abdomen. Another element influencing the determination of means as ordinary or extraordinary is the question of expense in relation to the individual's status.[114] Gury also holds the opinion that a maiden is excused from submitting to the treatment of a male doctor when her modesty causes her to fear this more than death itself.[115]

The teaching of Gury in the matter of the ordinary and extraordinary means of conserving life has been repeated substantially and most often verbatim by the authors who have produced editions of his work on moral theology.[116] However, there is a discussion in the Ballerini-Palmieri edition which is of considerable interest and significance. Relating the traditional teaching that intense pain would render a means extraordinary and that thus such operations as an amputation

---

nimis atroces afferente, vitam sibi servare; cum id sit extra communes vires positum. Eo in casu in communi aestimatione censetur justa de causa mortem tantummodo permittere." P. Scavini, *Theologia moralis universa* (Turin, 1865), II, n. 708.

[113] "Remediis extraordinariis, quaeque maximum dolorem afferant." J. Gury, *Compendium theologiae moralis*, 17th ed. (Rome, 1866), I, n. 391.

[114] Ordinary means "nec sumptus pro varia cuiusque conditione ingentes exposcunt." Ibid.

[115] "Non tenetur virgo operationem pati per manus medici, licet eius vita periclitetur, quando ea in re verecundia aequare potest aut etiam superare malum, quod morte pertimescitur." Ibid.

[116] See J. Gury, *Compendium theologiae moralis*, 14th ed., ed. A. Ballerini and D. Palmieri (Rome, 1907; hereafter Gury-Ballerini-Palmieri), I, nn. 389–391; J. Ferreres, *Compendium theologia moralis*, 16th ed. (Barcelona: Subirana, 1940), I, n. 489; and T. Jorio, *Theologia moralis*, 4th ed. (Naples: D'Auria, 1954), II, n. 165.

or incision into the abdomen would not be of obligation, Gury goes on to speculate a bit. If by some artificial means, it would be possible to induce sleep and thus relieve the pain, would the individual be bound to accept this type of sleep and submit to the operation. The answer is "as long as such inducing of sleep is a dangerous thing, certainly it is an extraordinary means: really, the very loss for some time of the use of reason and the mastery of his acts, such as occurs in this hypothesis, seems an extraordinary thing."[117]

It is very interesting to note this discussion, because it does not occur in the edition of Gury's *Compendium theologiae moralis* which was published with the help of Antonio Ballerini in 1866, the last year of Gury's life, and yet a somewhat similar discussion is found in the *Opus theologiae morale* of Ballerini, published posthumously by Domenico Palmieri. In a footnote in this latter work, the following is found:

> Theologians speak of the very bitter pains which an amputation produces. What if there is no pain because the senses have been put to sleep? Would it not be that the grave disadvantage of living with a mutilated body would just as readily excuse a sick man from undergoing the abscission as would the very harsh pains which last only a short while. This I leave for the learned to decide.[118]

In this period one begins to find reference to the new discovery of anesthesia. Anesthesia was somewhat known

---

[117] "Quamdiu talis immissio soporis sit res periculosa, certe este medium extra-ordinarium: verum vel ipsa amissio per aliquod tempus, usus rationis et dominii suorum actuum, qualis in hac hypothesi occurrit, res extraordinaria videtur." Gury-Ballerini-Palmieri, n. 391.

[118] "Theologi de acerbissimis doloribus, quos gignit amputatio, loquuntur. Quid, si nullus sit dolor propter sopitos sensus? Nonne grave imcommodum ducendi vitam cum corpore muti-

at the time. As regards its medical use, for all practical purposes, it was first successfully demonstrated in Boston, Massachusetts, in 1846.[119] The growing use of anesthesia did not have any world-shaking effect on the writings of the moralists. After a while, they began to acknowledge its advent and use, but they commented on it in terms which are obviously reserved and hesitant. The constant tradition of many years among so many great theologians had forced the moralists of this age to proceed carefully when faced with the numerous advances being made in the medical field.

In the two excerpts already cited, it can be seen that although there is recognition of the existence of anesthesia, doubt remains as to its safety.

Furthermore, even supposing that the use of anesthesia will be successful, the added difficulty of the temporary loss of the use of reason is mentioned. In the *Opus theologicum morale*, no doubt is left regarding the hesitancy insinuated there, even though it is disguised in question form. To submit to an amputation, whether it be performed painlessly or not, is too much to expect of any man, and therefore such surgery should not be classed as an ordinary means.[120] Except for this treatment, the work of Ballerini-Palmieri follows the traditional outline and, in fact, represents substantially the teaching of Busenbaum.

---

lato, tantumdem valet ad excusandum aegrum, ne abscissionem subeat, ac valent acerbissimi dolores brevi desituri? Id relinquo doctis definiendum?'"A. Ballerini, *Opus theologicum morale in Busenbaum medullam*, ed. D. Palmieri (Prati, 1899; hereafter Ballerini-Palmieri), II, p. 645, n. 868 note b.

[119]See D. Guthrie, "The History of Anaesthesia," in *A History of Medicine* (London: Nelson & Sons, 1947), pp. 301–306.

[120]Ballerini-Palmieri, II, p. 645, n. 868 note b.

Dr. Carl Capellmann (1841–1898), in his famous *Medicina pastoralis*, has a section titled "De operationibus vitae periculum afferentibus."[121] In this section, he discusses the lawfulness of dangerous operations, and also mentions the obligation of conserving one's life by these operations. He recalls the traditional teaching in the matter, namely, that the actual danger of surgical intervention renders these means extraordinary and therefore not obligatory. His source is St. Alphonsus. To this Capellmann replies,

> In this matter, I think one should note, however, that this opinion seems perhaps less appropriate because of the present standing of medicine and surgery, since difficult operations are performed now in circumstances entirely different and for the most part with greater success than before.[122]

Here full recognition of the progress of medical science is noted, and Capellmann is trying to apply the principles of moral theology to changed conditions. Immediately, then, he cites Gury and Scavini to show that the traditional teaching is that the excessive pain involved in a surgical operation renders such a means of conserving one's life extraordinary. Again Capellmann wonders whether anesthesia might put a different light on the subject. He asks,

> Does this resolve of probably escaping death, which otherwise would be certain, through an operation not painful in itself, exceed the ordinary strength of

---

[121] See C. Capellmann, *Medicina pastoralis*, 13th ed. (Aachen, 1901), pp. 24ss.

[122] "Qua in re advertendum tamen esse puto, hanc sententiam pro praesenti medicinae et chirurgiae sistu ideirco forte jam minus convenientem videri, quia operationes difficiles nunc circumstantiis plane mutatis ac plerumque meliori successu peraguntur quam antea." Ibid., p. 25.

men? It is sufficiently known even to the unskilled man that when chloroform is used, an operation can be performed without pain, and it can do much to lessen the anxiety and fear of a more difficult operation.[123]

Anticipating the objection that, even though anesthesia lessens or even eliminates pain during an operation, there will be pain after the anesthesia loses its effect, Capellmann answers that post-operative pains generally are not as intense as those during the operation, and for the most part are less than the pains arising from the disease which makes the operation necessary in the first place and which the individual will still have to suffer if he does not submit to the operation.[124] The deformity left by an operation is also not so cogent an excuse for not undergoing an operation as it was in earlier times, because technical remedies for the loss of a member are more advanced and offer a means of substitution.[125]

As advanced as Capellmann was in his thinking, however, he still was quite hesitant about being dogmatic in this matter—perhaps because of the long tradition to the contrary—and he ends the discussion with these words: "Therefore it seems that the opinion of theologians published up to now on this subject either could be or perhaps should

---

[123] Haeccine *voluntas*, cum aliqua probabiitate mortem certam operatione in se minime dolorosa effugiendi, communes hominum vires superat? Adhibito chloroformio operationem sine dolore perfici posse, etiam imperito jam satis compertum est, multumque valet ad demineundam anxietatem timoremque operationis difficilioris." Ibid., p. 26.

[124] Ibid.

[125] Etiam huic malo ars technica huius aetatis valde emendata levamen, atque saepius verum remedium praebet." Ibid.

be moderated. Certainly, however, I by no means intend to pass judgment on the matter."[126] The fact remains, however, that Capellmann was very impressed with the new use of anesthesia, and for him, at least, the whole moral aspect of surgical intervention had changed.[127] The next change that he could envision was the new application of the standard moral principles to the situation brought about by medical progress.

Augustin Lehmkuhl, S.J. (1834–1918), discusses the problem of the ordinary and extraordinary means of conserving life. This moralist mentions the traditional teaching in the matter and includes all the elements of extraordinary means which had been given by the preceding theologians. He cites the example of an amputation and recalls that the common teaching is that such an operation is not obligatory. Lehmkuhl admits that this teaching does not now enjoy the same favor with doctors and men of medicine as it once did, precisely because anesthesia can eliminate much of the pain previously connected with the procedure. However, Lehmkuhl insists that it is still not of obligation because, even if the element of pain were removed, the horror which would cause one to refuse the operation would still excuse from sin:

---

[126] Quapropter sententia theologorum de hac re hucusque vulgata videtur vel posse vel forte debere temperari. Equidem tamen rem diiudicare minime intendo." Ibid.

[127] "Nunc vero quomodo mutata sunt omnia! En aegrotum prorsus tranquillum sopore chloroformii, carentem dolore, libero voluntatis exercitio atque renisu. Perfecta cum quiete operatio firmiter ac diigenter perfici potest, aegrotus autem expergefactus, quum dolor pro rerum circumstantiis sit exiguus, non laborat nisi ex effectibus soporis chloroformii raro molestioribus. Quod sane miseris aegrotis magni est momenti magnumque beneficium." Ibid., p. 41.

> Even now, I think scarcely is a mortal sin commit-
> ted by the one who, terrified of an amputation,
> refuses to submit to it. ... One should not omit the
> fact that not the torments alone, which partly can
> be deadened now, but also great horror can be the
> reason why it would be licit to refuse a great opera-
> tion—I am not speaking now, e.g., of cutting off a
> finger and its joint.[128]

It is the opinion of Lehmkuhl, therefore, that the advent of
anesthesia had not eliminated all the elements of extraordinary
means, and therefore one should proceed carefully before
imposing as a moral obligation a procedure which under one
aspect or another has enjoyed considerable progress, even
success, in the medical field.

The writings of Cardinal José Vives y Tuto, O.F.M. Cap.,
and Canon J. B. Pighi adhere closely to tradition. These
authors list as examples of extraordinary means the amputation of a leg and the surgical operation which appears to a
virgin more terrifying than death itself.[129]

Gustavus Waffelaert (1837–1931) follows de Lugo quite
closely in his treatment of the ordinary and extraordinary means
of conserving life.[130] The ordinary means are of obligation and

---

[128] "Mortale peccatum etiam nunc vix committi puto ab eo,
qui amputationem multum horrens eam pati detrectet ... tamen
omitti non debet, non cruciatus solos, qui ex pane sopiri nunc
possunt, sed etiam horrorem magnum pro ratione haberi posse,
cur magna operationem—non enim loquor v. g. de digito ejusque
articulo abscindendo—detrectari liceat." Lehmkuhl, *Theologia
moralis*, I, p. 345.

[129] See J. Vives y Tuto, *Compendium theologiae moralis*, 9th
ed. (Rome: Pustet, 1909), n. 308; J. Pighi, *Cursus theologiae moralis*
(Verona, 1901), III, n. 180. See also in this matter C. Marc and
F. X. Gestermann, *Institutiones morales alphonsianae*, ed. J. Raus,
18th ed. (Lyon, 1927), I, n. 754; and Aertnys-Damen, *Theologiae
moralis*, I, n. 566.

the extraordinary means are not. What are the ordinary means? Waffelaert replies that "they do not consist 'in individibili' but must be determined from the various considerations indicated in the proposition and finally, the matter must be settled in a determined event from moral judgment."[131]

Januarius Bucceroni, S.J. (1841–1918), says that extraordinary means lie outside the limits of common endurance.[132] Therefore, a sick person must take only ordinary medications and need not spend great sums of money or employ unusual remedies.[133] Likewise, Achille Vander Heeren writes in 1912 that an individual is bound "to make use of all the ordinary means which are indicated in the usual course of things."[134] However, one is not bound "to employ remedies which, considering one's condition, are regarded as extraordinary and involving extraordinary expenditure."[135]

Vermeersch does not depart from tradition either. He is content with mentioning the usual examples of extraordinary means.[136] This is, in general, true also of Joseph Ubach, S.J.,

---

[130] See G. Waffelaert, *De virtutibus cardinalibus* (Bruges, 1886), vol. II, *De justitia*, nn. 39ss.

[131] "Media illa ordinaria non consistant in individibili, sed ex variis considerationibus in propositione indicates sint dimetienda et denique tandem ex morali judicio sit in determinato eventu res absolvenda." Ibid., n. 43.

[132] "Et sane media extraordinaria extra communes vires posita sunt." J. Bucceroni, *Institutiones theologiae moralis*, 6th ed. (Rome, 1914–1915), I, n. 715.

[133] Ibid, n. 716.

[134] A. Vander Heeren, "Suicide," *The Catholic Encyclopedia* (New York, Appleton Co., 1912), XIV, p. 327. See also *Dictionnaire de Théologie Catholique* (Paris: Letouzey et Ané, 1941), tom. 14, col. 2748.

[135] Vander Heeren, "Suicide."

[136] See Vermeersch, *Theologia moralis*, II, n. 300.

although he is inclined to go a bit further. For example, Ubach[137] lists vehement pain, danger of death, extraordinary expenditure of money, and great fear as elements which make a surgical operation an extraordinary means. Pain, he says, is generally removed by anesthesia; extraordinary cost is often absent because a surgical operation is usually performed in a public hospital. Fear frequently is not present and, if it were, one should try to eliminate it if it is irrational. However, if considerable fear of the operation remains, then this would be a legitimate excuse from undergoing it. Ubach is quite reserved, however, when treating danger of death. Much has been said, he feels, to extol the progress made in the medical field, but he emphasizes that one must never forget that an element of danger still exists and this can render such an operation extraordinary and thus not obligatory. He then makes the statement that "since some one of these reasons is not usually lacking, ordinarily a major surgical operation is not obligatory."[138]

The treatment found in Hieronymus Noldin, S.J., and Albert Schmitt, S.J. (1940)[139] is quite good. It is precise and to the point. After stating that extraordinary means are not usually of obligation, these authors note that extraordinary means should be determined from the common estimate of men. Those who are gravely sick and refuse to employ the services of a doctor and abide by his advice, when this can be done easily and when there is hope of recovery, are guilty of sin. However, any remedy that is very costly, considering

---

[137] See J. Ubach, *Theologia moralis* (Buenos Aires: Sociedad San Miguel, 1935), I, n. 488.

[138] "Quare, cum aliqua ex hix causis conseuverit non deese, ordinarie magna operatio chirurgica non est obligatoria." Ibid.

[139] See Noldin-Schmitt, *Summa theologiae moralis*, II, pp. 307–308

one's status, or very painful and thus difficult is not obligatory. Since a remedy that is very costly is not of obligation,
would a rich man be bound to employ it if he could afford
to pay for it? Noldin and Schmitt answer that not even a rich
man would be bound to employ the services of very skilled
doctors or to leave his home in order to seek a better climate.
This is true because "all these means are extraordinary."[140]
Hence, it can be seen that these authors feel that there is a
definite limit beyond which a remedy should be considered
extraordinary, absolutely speaking.[141]

Regarding major surgical operations or a major amputation, Noldin and Schmitt are rather definite.[142] They recognize that the older moralists excused an individual from
submitting to these operations. However, since many of the
elements on which these moralists based their reasoning
have now been eliminated, it seems that such operations
should be called obligatory. Anesthesia has removed pain.
Operations now enjoy much greater success, and artificial
substitutes for natural limbs have been perfected. Two conditions are posited by these authors, however, before such
an operation can be called obligatory. First, there must be a
great probability that certain danger of death will be avoided.

---

[140] "Quia haec omnia extrordinaria sunt." Ibid., p. 308

[141] See E. Healy, *Moral Guidance*, p. 162. In an example, Father
Healy suggests two thousand dollars as an absolute norm—an
amount that even a rich man would not be obliged to spend.
Extraordinary means for this author are those means which "exceed
the normal strength of men in general." See also E. Genicot and
I. Salsmans, *Institutiones theologiae moralis*, 17th ed. (Brussels:
L'Edition Universelle, 1951; hereafter Genicot-Salsmans), I, n. 364,
where one reads "vim pecuniae ingentem expendere, nemo, etiam
ditissimus, tenetur, etiamsi aliter vitam protrahere nequeat."

[142] See Noldin-Schmitt, *Summa theologiae moralis*, II,
pp. 307–308.

Second, there should not be any intense subjective horror of the operation present.[143]

A somewhat similar treatment of surgical operations is found in Edouard Génicot, S.J., and Joseph Salsmans, S.J. (1941).[144] They state that even when a major surgical operation can be performed without tremendous pain or great danger, it would be difficult to say that *per se* such an operation is obligatory when vehement subjective horror is present. Certainly this horror would produce an extraordinary difficulty.[145] Furthermore, they feel that often a prudent doubt remains especially in regard to the enduring success of major operations. These authors do suggest, however, that an individual should rid himself of any exaggerated fear of operations and, generally speaking, consent to them when it is necessary for the conservation of his life.[146]

Benoît Henri Merkelbach, O.P. (1871–1942), excuses a man from employing "extraordinary, choice, unusual, more costly and very difficult means,"[147] in order to recover his health. These, he says, are not obligatory because the law demanding one to "protract"[148] his life does not oblige him at the cost of such great trouble.[149] Today, however, Merkelbach notes, many operations which in days gone by were quite difficult and dangerous are now performed very easily and

---

[143] Ibid.

[144] See Genicot-Salsmans, *Institutiones*, n. 364.

[145] Ibid.

[146] Ibid.

[147] "Media extraordinaria, exquisita, inusitata, pretiosiora, valde difficilia." B. Merkelbach, *Summa theologiae moralis* (Paris: Desclée, 1935), II, n. 353.

[148] "Protrahendi." Ibid.

[149] "Cum tanto incommode." Ibid.

safely. Therefore, it can be said that "they have now become ordinary means."[150]

In treating this very point, Ludovicus Fanfani, O.P. (1876–1955), uses the same words as Merkelbach except that he concludes this way: "Therefore operations of this type cannot always be called extraordinary means."[151] It is interesting to note this, because the very same idea is expressed in just slightly different terms; they are different enough, however, to make one realize that Fanfani is a bit more hesitant about stating categorically that a modern surgical operation is now an ordinary means.

In his *Moral and Pastoral Theology* (1938), Henry Davis, S.J., is content to say that a man must preserve his life by the use of ordinary means. He is not bound, however, to employ "extraordinary expensive methods nor methods that would inflict on him almost intolerable pain or shame."[152]

In his doctoral dissertation, *The Morality of Organic Transplantation* (1944), Bert Cunningham, C.M., says, "Man's custody of his own body demands that he conserve his life by every reasonable means, for that is in agreement with his position as custodian of the life given to him by God."[153]

Marcelino Zalba, S.J. requires a man to use only congruous and common means and ordinary diligence.[154] There

---

[150] "Ac ita jam facta sunt media ordinaria." Ibid.

[151] "Ideoque huiusmodi operationes nequeunt semper dici media extraordinaria." Fanfani, *Manuale theorico-practicale*, II, n. 225, dub. I. See also Fanfani's other references to ordinary and extraordinary means at nn. 88 and 169.

[152] H. Davis, *Moral and Pastoral Theology*, 3rd ed. (London: Sheed and Ward, 1938), II, p. 141.

[153] B. Cunningham, *The Morality of Organic Transplantation* (Washington, D.C.: Catholic University Press, 1944), pp. 95–96.

is no obligation to use extraordinary means or extraordinary diligence except *per accidens*.[155] In applying the principle, Zalba feels that one would not be bound "to undergo a very dangerous operation or a very troublesome convalescence."[156] Neither is a person bound to suffer the extraordinary pain of a surgical operation "if, however, this case ever occurs supposing modern methods."[157] It is interesting to take cognizance of the fact that Zalba recognizes that a period of recovery can be very harsh and thus be an extraordinary means. His opinion about the moral obligations involved in modern operations is guarded, as the reader can see. Perhaps he does not want to state definitively that many major operations today are ordinary means, as Merkelbach did.

In the latest edition of Antonio Lanza and Pietro Palazzini's *Theologia moralis* (1955), one reads that what at another time was held to be an extraordinary means has today, on account of the progress of science, perhaps become ordinary.[158] What means are extraordinary? This should be decided in individual cases. However, it must be kept in

---

[154] "Media congrua; sed per se solum communia ... et per ordinariam diligentiam." Regatillo-Zalba, *Theologiae moralis*, II, n. 254.

[155] "Per accidens tamen potest aliquis teneri ad media extraordinaria applicanda vel ad extraordinariam diligentiam abhibendam." Ibid.

[156] "Neque operationi valde periculose vel convalescentiae molestissimae se submittere." Ibid., n. 254, applicatio 3.

[157] "Si tamen casus iste eveniat unquam suppositis mediis hodiernis." Ibid.

[158] "Quod alias ut medium extraordinarium habebatur, hodie, ob scientiae progressum, forte ordinarium factum est." A. Lanza and P. Palazzini, *Theologia moralis* (Turin: Marietti, 1955; hereafter Lanza-Palazzini), II, n. 125.

mind that in ordinary circumstances, no one is obliged to undergo a "grave inconvenience" to conserve his life.[159]

The shorter manuals of moral theology are in great measure synopses of the teaching already recorded here as regards the doctrine on the ordinary and extraordinary means of conserving life. Adolphe Tanquerey, S.S., mentions that one need not prolong his life with great inconvenience.[160] Neither is an individual bound to undergo a dangerous or very painful or greatly displeasing operation.[161] Antonio Arregui gives the same doctrine.[162]

However, Heribert Jone, O.F.M. Cap., is inclined to be a little more specific. He exempts even wealthy people from the necessity of going to a far-distant place or health resort. Even the wealthy would not be obliged to summon the best-known physicians. It is the opinion of these authors also that no one is gravely obliged to undergo a major surgical operation except *per accidens*, and even then the success of the operation must be morally certain.[163]

One of the few modern theologians to afford any special treatment of the problem of the ordinary and extraordinary means of conserving life is Gerald Kelly, S.J.

---

[159] "Obligatio subeundi grave incommodum ad ipsum servandum non probatur." Ibid.

[160] "Lex enim diu vitam protrahendi non obligat cum tanto incommodo." A. Tanquerey, *Synopsis theologiae moralis et pastoralis* (Paris: Desclée & Socii, 1953), III, p. 248.

[161] "Nec quisquam obligatur periculosam aut valde dolorosam vel maxime displicentem operationem subire." Ibid.

[162] "Non autem necessario mediis extraordinariis, sc. pro sua condicione valde sumptuosis, vel dolore aut pudore nimis arduis." A. Arregui, *Summarium theologiae moralis*, 18th ed. (Bilbao: Mensajero, 1948), n. 234.

[163] See H. Jone, *Moral Theology*, 8th ed., trans. U. Adelman, (Westminister, MD: Newman Press, 1948), n. 210.

His writings will be looked at more closely in succeeding chapters of this dissertation. Suffice it to say now that these writings are of definite importance because of his experience and skill in treating medico-moral problems and because of his realization of the practical import of the problem of the ordinary and extraordinary means of conserving life in modern medical procedure.[164]

This chapter has included the opinions the most noteworthy moral theologians regarding the means of conserving life. It is with this teaching in mind that in the next chapter an attempt will be made to study more closely the nature of the ordinary and extraordinary means. In this way, it is hoped that the entire study will be based on traditional teaching. While it is true that theologians of past ages perhaps never imagined the almost miraculous progress of medical science which is so well known today, they nonetheless left behind them the basic principles whereby even the moral problems of modern medicine can be solved correctly.

---

[164] See G. Kelly, "The Duty of Using Artificial Means of Preserving Life," *Theological Studies* 11 (June 1950), pp. 203–220; "The Duty to Preserve Life," *Theological Studies* 12 (December 1951), pp. 550–556; and *Medico-Moral Problems* (St. Louis: Catholic Hospital Association of the U.S. and Canada, 1954), V, pp. 6–15. Another treatment of considerable import is J. Paquin, *Morale et medécine* (Montreal: L'Immaculée-Conception, 1955), pp. 398–403.

Chapter 3

OBLIGATION IN CHOICE OF MEANS

In the previous chapters, we have presented a discussion of the basic duty of conserving one's life and a report of the opinions of the most noteworthy moral theologians in regard to the ordinary and extraordinary means of conserving life.

The nature of the ordinary and extraordinary means of conserving life and the moral obligation of using these means are the subjects of the present chapter. In determining the nature of these means, of necessity we shall look more closely at the opinions already presented in chapter 2. An analysis of the writings of the theologians will give the elements by which we can determine more precisely the nature of the ordinary and extraordinary means of conserving life. These theologians as a rule did not define the terms "ordinary and extraordinary means of conserving life," but they did describe the means and they did underline the elements which constitute them.

Once we have determined the nature of the ordinary and extraordinary means of conserving life, we shall discuss in the second section of this chapter the moral obligation of using them and the extent to which this obligation binds.

In this section, we intend to gather from the writings of the moralists the elements which they consider essential to the concept of the ordinary and extraordinary means of conserving life. We shall then study the implications in these elements and thus be able to determine the nature of ordinary and extraordinary means. However, prior to this it will be profitable to discuss some preliminary notions.

PRELIMINARY NOTIONS

Natural and Artificial Means

One of the first distinctions which we find made in this matter by the moralists is the one in which the natural means of conserving life are distinguished from the artificial means. In this present discussion, we are using the word *artificial* to designate a means which is devised and made by man for the conservation of his life. A *natural means* is a means which nature itself provides for the conservation of man's life. The older moralists used the term "natural means." They did not, however, use the term "artificial means," but usually they described an artificial means in a negative way by pointing out that such a means is not a natural means. We have seen this already in the writings of Vitoria: "A similar case does not exist between food and drugs. For food is *per se* a means ordered to the life of the animal and it is natural, drugs are not."[1] Vitoria wants to emphasize that a man is not obliged to use every possible means of conserving his life but that, basically, his obligation begins only with those means that are natural and intended by nature for the conservation of man's life: "A man is not held to employ all the possible

---

[1] "Quod non est simile de pharamaco et alimento. Alimentum enim per se est medium ordinatum ad vitam animalis et naturale, non autem pharmacum." Vitoria, *De temperantia*, n.1.

means of conserving his life, but the means which are *per se* intended for that purpose."[2] Fundamentally, there is a clear distinction in the mind of Vitoria between natural means of conserving life and artificial means. It would seem also that he would say that natural means are obligatory and artificial means are not obligatory. In any event, he definitely assigns a stricter moral obligation of employing natural means than of employing artificial means of conserving life.

Reading further in this same section of Vitoria's writings, we note an apparent contradiction to what has just been stated. Vitoria proposes the situation in which a person would have moral certitude that if he should take a certain medicine, he would regain his health; if he refuses to take the medicine, he will die. Is he obliged to take the medicine? Vitoria seems to reply that he is bound to use the medicine, and that if he does not take it, "he really does not seem to be excused from mortal sin."[3] The reasons for this answer are, first of all, that this same person would be required to give the medicine to a sick neighbor; otherwise he would be guilty of sin. Secondly, Vitoria says, "Medicine *per se* also is intended by nature for health."[4]

Hence, we see that Vitoria apparently is saying that drugs and medicines are not obligatory because they are not natural means intended by nature for the conservation of man's life and saying also in the same section that drugs and medicines are *per se* intended by nature for health and are obligatory. There is no doubt that an apparent contradiction

---

[2] "Nec tenetur homo adhibere omnia media possibilia ad conservandam vitam, sed media per se ad hoc ordinate." Ibid.

[3] "Non videtur profecto excusari a mortali." Ibid.

[4] "Medicina per se etiam ordinate est ad salutem a natura." Ibid.

exists. However, it would seem that a correct understanding of Vitoria's words can come only from an understanding of the entire context. Recall that he said that the case existing between food and drugs is not a similar one. This is true. Food is primarily intended by nature for the basic sustenance of animal life. Food for man is basically and fundamentally necessary from the very beginning of his temporal existence. It is basically required by his human life, and nature intends food for this purpose. That is why man has the right to grow food and kill animals. Furthermore, because it is a law of nature that man sustain himself by food, it is a duty for man to nourish himself by food.

In the case of drugs and medicines, the same is not true. Drugs and medicines are intended *per se* by nature to help man conserve his life. However, this is by way of exception. Drugs and medicines are not the basic way by which man is to nourish his life. They are intended by nature to aid man in the conservation of his life when he is sick or in pain or unable to sustain himself by natural means. These artificial means are not natural means, but they are intended by nature to help man protect, sustain, and conserve his life. If man were never to be sick, he would never need medicines. If he is sick, however, it is quite *natural* for him to make use of *artificial* means of *conserving* his life.

Vitoria is correct, therefore, in making a clear distinction between natural means of conserving life and artificial means of conserving life. He is also correct when he explains that natural means, such as food, are intended *per se* by nature for the conservation of man's life, whereas artificial means are intended *per se* by nature for this same purpose but as a means of supplementing the natural means when this becomes necessary.

In regard to the obligation of using natural means of conserving life, Vitoria clearly states that the natural means are obligatory. With regard to the obligation of employing the artificial means of conserving life, his teaching again appears contradictory. In one place he seems to say that artificial means are not obligatory; in another place, he clearly states that there is a moral obligation to employ them when necessary for the conservation of one's life. In this particular matter also, an understanding of what Vitoria means to imply will render his actual words more understandable.

Vitoria's statement that an artificial means is *per se* intended by nature for the health of a person is quite understandable. It is also clear that Vitoria makes the use of artificial means a matter of obligation when the physical condition of the individual requires it. We must recall, however, that Vitoria is positing a condition in this matter. He states in his proposed case that the individual concerned has moral certitude that a medicine will bring him health. Further on in the same discussion, he actually admits that the possession beforehand of moral certitude of benefit deriving from the use of medicines is not obligatory. His words are, "But since this rarely can be certain, therefore they are not to be condemned with mortal sin who have declared universally an abstinence from drugs."[5]

We can see, therefore, that the teaching of Vitoria in this matter is that medicines and drugs—in fact artificial means in general—are intended by nature to supplement the natural means of conserving life. They are intended to help man to conserve his life when the use of merely natural means, such as food, sunshine, rest, etc., are not sufficient because of the individual's physical condition. As such, therefore, the artificial means are obligatory. However, in Vitoria's time, the development and progress of medical

---

[5] "Sed quia hoc vix potest esse certum, ideo non sunt damnandi de mortali, qui in universum decreverunt abstinere a pharmacis." Ibid.

helps to conserving life had not reached the point where their use would give any sure hope of benefit. One could not have moral certitude of benefit. Hence, Vitoria is quite logical and quite correct in not demanding that a person is under obligation to use these artificial means.

To summarize Vitoria's teaching in this matter, we may say that natural means of conserving life are *per se* intended by nature as the means whereby a man is to conserve his life, and ordinarily these are strictly obligatory. Furthermore, artificial means of conserving life are *per se* intended by nature as a means whereby man can supplement the natural means of conserving life when these natural means are lacking or insufficient. Ordinarily, these artificial means are obligatory too if they can be obtained and used conveniently and with some certitude of benefit.

Sayrus makes the very same distinction. In fact, it is interesting to note that he uses Vitoria's very words in this section.[6] Actually, all he has done has been to repeat verbatim Vitoria's argument. One notion, however, is his own. He adds the term "naturally produced" to the expression "common foods": "No one in order to prolong his life is bound to use the best and more delicate foods, even though he be able; he need use only the common ones, naturally produced."[7] Here again, the same reasoning that motivated Vitoria in this matter is apparent in the writings of Sayrus. Basically, he feels that only what is a natural means of conserving life is obligatory. He repeats the case, which was proposed by Vitoria, about the necessary use of medicine, and we can see

---

[6] Sayrus, *Clavis regia casuum conscientae*, lib. VII, cap. IX, n. 28.

[7] "Nemo ad vitam prolongandam, cibis optimis et delicatioribus uti tenetur, etiamsi posit, sed communibus naturaliter productis." Ibid.

that Sayrus also is influenced by the condition of the medical science of his day. One cannot be sure of success in the use of medicines; therefore, they can hardly be called obligatory. However, the use of medicines would be obligatory if one could be sure that they would be of benefit.

Sánchez also says that one would not be bound to use medicines to prolong one's life, such as taking a drug for many years to avoid fevers.[8] He also uses the expression "means directed by nature for sustenance."[9] It would seem that Sánchez does not oblige a person to make use of a drug for many years in order to avoid a fever not because the use of a drug could never be obligatory but because the use of a drug for many years is not obligatory.

When one reads the writings of these older moralists in the whole context, one understands rather easily why they are eager on the one hand to term medicines a means of conserving life directly intended by nature for the purpose of conserving life, and therefore obligatory when necessary, and why, on the other hand, these same authors seem willing to contradict themselves. As the success of medicine became more certain, the authors wrote differently. For example, Tamburini writes that one is bound to use only "ordinary foods *per se* intended to conserve life."[10] Then he says in the same section that one is not obliged to take very costly and extraordinary medicines, "since it is sufficient

---

[8] "Non tenetur quis uti medicinis ad prolongandam vitam ... ut quotannis sumere pharmacum ad vitandas bebres etc." Sánchez, *Consilia seu opuscula moralia*, tom. II, lib. V, cap. I, dub. 33, n. 4.

[9] "Mediis ordinatis a natura ad sustentationem." Ibid., n. 11.

[10] "Non tenetur quis uti cibis nisi ordinariis per se ordinatis ad vitam conservandam." Tamburini, *Explicatio decalogi*, lib. VI, cap. II, sect. II, n. 11.

to use common medicines."[11] Here we can see clearly that while the term *"per se* intended"is used for ordinary foods and these are obligatory, yet in the same section Tamburini calls common medicines obligatory.

In the writings of the previous authors there is hesitancy about stating any obligation even in regard to the use of common medicines. Hence, we can appreciate that the moral teaching of the older moralists in this matter is quite solid, even though in their writings they would seem to confuse principle and practice. *In principle*, artificial means of conserving life are obligatory; but for these authors, *in practice*, these means are not obligatory because of some circumstance which eliminates the duty of using them. For example, the medicines are too costly or they do not provide any serious hope of benefit. This seems to be the reason why in one and the same context an author will require the use of artificial means, and then say that these means are not of obligation.

What these older moralists were actually saying can be well explained by the terms "ordinary and extraordinary means of conserving life." When these moralists were living, artificial means of conserving life were extraordinary means because they were too costly or did not offer any hope of benefit. When, however, medicines became useful and offered some hope of success, these means became ordinary means, and the moralists then called them obligatory. It does not seem, therefore, that the writings of the older moralists provide any argument for the opinion that artificial means of conserving life are never obligatory. When one understands the meaning in these writings, one will see

---

[11] "Cum satis sit medicinis uti communibus." Ibid.

that these moralists in principle do oblige a person to make use of artificial means of conserving life when these means are truly ordinary means. They seem to make the distinction between natural and artificial means because natural means generally were ordinary means and thus obligatory, whereas artificial means in this period of history were usually for one reason or another extraordinary means.

God intends the development of science for the good of man. When science can provide a means of conserving man's life which can be a supplement to a natural means, then this artificial means would seem to be obligatory. It is true, however, that whereas natural means in general are ordinary means, artificial means of conserving life can quite often be extraordinary means and thus not obligatory. When artificial means are ordinary means, then they are obligatory. We will see more closely, as this chapter progresses, the conditions required in determining a means as ordinary or extraordinary. The object of this discussion so far has been to show that the terms "artificial means" and "extraordinary means" are not coextensive. An artificial means can be an ordinary means of conserving life.

As a final point, we may point out that an artificial means of conserving life can be either a cure for a disease, such as a medicine, or a means of supplanting a natural means of sustaining life, such as intravenous feeding. This distinction would not seem to change either in theory or in practice the teaching mentioned here. If the artificial means, whether a cure or a substitution for a natural means of conserving life, is an ordinary means, it is obligatory. It is for this reason that in mentioning artificial means we have referred to them as means of supplementing the natural means of conserving life, intending thereby to include in the term "artificial means" both the means of curing a disease and means which supplant a natural function.

Ordinary Means versus
Ordinary Medical Procedures

The distinction existing between the expressions *ordinary means of conserving life* and *ordinary medical procedures* is a very interesting and important one. It is particularly important in any practical question concerning the duty of employing an artificial means, because there is danger of confusing the terms. In point of fact, an ordinary medical procedure is not necessarily an ordinary means of conserving life. What is an ordinary treatment in medical procedure can easily be a means of conserving life which the moralist will not term either ordinary or obligatory. [12] The moralists of past ages had no need of making this distinction, because most medical and surgical procedures were admittedly extraordinary means. Today, however, men are more conscious of the wonders of medical progress, and they are more accustomed to employing medical and surgical remedies. Therefore, it is easy to imagine that what is surely ordinary as a medical procedure might appear ordinary also as a morally obligatory means of conserving life. However, such a case is not necessarily true. For example, a surgical intervention is an ordinary medical procedure today in case of acute appendicitis. It probably is also morally an ordinary means of conserving life in most instances. However, for some individuals, it still could be an extraordinary means due to some unusual set of circumstances. Thus it would not be obligatory. The expense involved in the operation or the lack of proper medi-

---

[12] "La difficulté consiste a préciser le sens de ces deux expressions: remèdes ou traitements ordinaires, remèdes ou traitements extrordinaires. Le langue médical appellera traitements ordinaires ceux qui sont habituellement employés pour telle ou telle maladie; mais, au point de vue theologique, de tels traitements peuvent parfois etre extraordinares." Paquin, *Morale et medicine*, p. 398.

cal and surgical facilities could easily render the operation an extraordinary means for a particular individual. It is true that usually an extraordinary medical procedure will also be an extraordinary means of conserving life. However, it is well to understand from the beginning of this discussion that an ordinary medical remedy is not necessarily an obligatory ordinary means of conserving life.

The Common Elements

We have noted above that this study of the nature of the ordinary means of conserving life will be founded on the elements derived from an analysis of the writings of the moral theologians. This will be true also of the study of the nature of the extraordinary means of conserving life, which will be found in a succeeding section of this chapter.

In order that the elements involved in these terms may be seen more clearly, a table of moral theologians and the elements which they include in their discussions of the means of conserving life appears on the following pages. The table is by no means exhaustive, but it is representative and can be of assistance in conveying the frequency with which some elements are mentioned in the theological discussions of the ordinary and extraordinary means of conserving life. There are other elements mentioned by the moralists which have not been noted in the table because they have not been common to many authors. Where, however, there is need of mentioning such elements, proper citation is made in the text itself. It is also well to note that in the table the terms appear in Latin. (English equivalents appear in the notes to the table.) Usually the exact Latin expression is common to all the designated authors. Occasionally, however, an author may have used a different expression or a different language

continued on page 122

Ordinary and Extraordinary Means in the Writings of the Major Moral Theologians

Author	Ordinary Means					Extraordinary Means								
	1	2	3	4	5	6	7	8	9	10	11	12	13	14
Vitoria	×	×				×	×		×	×	×			
Soto									×		×			
Molina	×										×			
Sayrus	×	×				×	×		×	×	×			×
Banez	×	×	×								×	×	×	
Sánchez				×										×
Lessius				×					×		×			
Bonacina				×							×			
Laymann				×						×				
Gabr. a SV									×		×			
De Lugo	×	×		×							×	×		×
Diana									×		×			
Tournely				×		×			×	×	×	×		
Salmantic.	×									×	×	×	×	×
Busenbaum	×							×			×		×	×
Escobar												×		
Tamburini		×					×		×		×			
Holzmann				×							×			
Sporer			×	×					×	×				
Reiffenstuel	×	×	×	×			×			×				
Lacroix	×			×				×			×			×
Roncaglia		×									×	×	×	
Mazzotta	×						×			×				×
Elbel		×	×							×				

NOTES: Numbers indicate means mentioned by the authors whose names are marked with an ×, as follows: **Ordinary means** are (1) *spes salutis*, hope of benefit; (2) *media communia*, means commonly used; (3) *secundum proportionem status*, current status factor; (4) *non difficilia*, means that are not too difficult; and (5) *facilia*, reasonably simple means. **Extraordinary means** are (6) *quaedam impossibilitas*, a certain impossibility factor; (7) *summus*

120

Ordinary and Extraordinary Means, *continued*

Author	Ordinary Means					Extraordinary Means								
	1	2	3	4	5	6	7	8	9	10	11	12	13	14
Billuart	×	×	×	×							×			
Patuzzi	×				×	×	×			×	×			
Alphonsus	×							×					×	
Scavini								×				×	×	
Gury		×								×	×			
Ballerini-P.	×							×				×	×	
Pighi											×			
Lehmkuhl			×	×					×	×			×	
Marc-Gest.						×		×			×		×	
Waffelaert	×			×	×									
Bucceroni	×	×								×		×		×
Ferreres		×								×	×			
Vander Heer.		×								×	×			
Genicot-Sals.			×	×		×				×		×	×	
Noldin-Schm.	×		×	×	×					×		×	×	
Aertnys-Dam.			×	×		×				×				
Vermeersch								×			×		×	×
Ubach		×				×				×		×	×	
Merkelbach		×	×			×				×	×			×
Davis										×	×			
Jone	×													
Zalba		×	×									×		
Kelly	×		×			×				×		×	×	
Paquin	×		×									×	×	

labor, greatest effort required; (8) *nimis dura*, excessive hardship factor; (9) *quidam cruciatus*, a certain excruciating pain; (10) *sumptus extraordinarius*, extraordinary expenditure; (11) *media pretiosa*, high-priced means; (12) *ingens dolor*, excessive pain; (13) *vehemens horror*, intense fear/repugnance; and (14) *media exquisita*, the very best means. Bullets indicate means mentioned in the author's works, which can be found in the bibliography.

to connote the same idea. His name is marked, nonetheless, as having used the more common phrase.

The reader will note that we are going to discuss separately the nature of the ordinary means of conserving life and the nature of the extraordinary means. Although this method is not common in the treatises found in the moral theology books, we feel that to separate the two discussions will better emphasize the difference between the two terms.

The Nature of Ordinary Means

Hope of Benefit
(*Spes salutis*)

It is clear from the writings of the moralists that a means of conserving life must offer *some hope of a beneficial result* before such a means can be termed ordinary and obligatory. Vitoria speaks of the obligation that a sick man has to take food or nourishment if he can take it "with a certain hope of life."[13] Further on in the same writing, he says that a man who has moral certitude that he can regain his health by the use of a drug is bound to use the drug.[14] After Vitoria, this notion of a hope of benefit in the question of the ordinary means of conserving life was repeated by many moral theologians.

The teaching that an ordinary means of conserving life must offer a hope of benefit is certainly in harmony with common sense. It would be unreasonable to bind an individual with a moral obligation of employing a remedy or cure which offers no hope of benefit. All theologians agree to this, although not all moralists actually mention it in their discussions of the ordinary and extraordinary means

---

[13] "Cum aliqua spe vitae." Vitoria, *De temperantia*, n. 1.
[14] Ibid.

of conserving life. No one, however, writes in opposition to this teaching.

The question of more practical import is how much hope of benefit a means must offer before it can be called an ordinary means. We have mentioned in chapter 2 the case cited by de Lugo, in which a man is condemned to death by fire.[15] Surrounded by flames, the man notices that he has sufficient water to extinguish some of the fire but not all of it. De Lugo notes that the man concerned is not morally obligated to use the water, because he cannot extinguish the flames once and for all and thus escape death. If he could extinguish the fire, he would be obliged to do so. However, he is not obliged merely to postpone his death by extinguishing part of the fire. In other words, the element of benefit is introduced. The means and remedies employed, even though in themselves common means, must offer some hope of benefit or help to the conservation of life before they become obligatory ordinary means. The benefit to be derived from the use of these means must be worthwhile. It must be worthwhile in quality and duration. Furthermore, it must be worthwhile in consideration of the effort expended in using the means. In a word, the use of a means must offer a *proportionate* hope of benefit or else it is not an ordinary means.

Hence we can see that a means of conserving life, even though it be a very common remedy, cannot be termed an ordinary means if it offers little or no hope of benefit. The fact that a means very definitely gives hope of some benefit but not a hope of proportionate benefit in no way charges the case. A hope of little benefit is to be considered morally as nothing. De Lugo phrases this doctrine in the following manner: "The obligation of conserving life by ordinary means is not

---

[15] De Lugo, *De justitia et jure*, disp. X, sect. I, n. 30.

an obligation of using these means for such a brief conservation—which is morally considered as nothing at all."[16]

De Lugo clearly states that any means which is to be employed for the conservation of one's life must give definite hope of being proportionately useful and beneficial before it can be called obligatory. It is noteworthy that de Lugo applies this doctrine even to the taking of food,[17] which is a purely natural means of conserving life. In other words, for de Lugo, any means, whether natural or artificial, must give proportionate hope of success and benefit; otherwise, it is not an ordinary means and is thus not obligatory. Gerald Kelly, commenting on those words of de Lugo, writes, "It may be that the principle, *parum pro nihilo reputatur*, is really contained in the preceding principle, *nemo ad inutile tenetur*. Yet there seems to be a slight difference. Furthermore, de Lugo applies his principle even to the taking of food, which is a purely natural means of preserving life, whereas the other authors were speaking only of remedies for illness."[18]

Closely allied to this notion of proportionate hope of benefit is the element of danger which many recent authors mention in connection with their discussion of modern remedies and treatment. The earlier moralists were cognizant of the same element of danger, and that is why they spoke so clearly on the notion of proportionate benefit. In other words, a remedy or treatment must give definite and proportionate hope of success. If a procedure does not offer this proportionate hope of success, it is clearly not an ordinary means. It is true that as medical science has progressed,

----

[16] "Obligatio conservandi vitam per media ordinaria, non est obligatio utendi mediis ad illam brevem conservationem, quae moraliter pro nihilo reputatur." Ibid.

[17] Ibid.

[18] Kelly, "The Duty of Using Artificial Means," p. 208.

many surgical operations and medical treatments that were dangerous and offered no proportionate hope of success have been perfected. Since they are not usually dangerous now, and do give hope of success and benefit, they have become ordinary means, at least in regard to the element of success and benefit.

If a medical procedure involves risk or danger and does not at the same time offer proportionate hope of success, the procedure is not morally obligatory. This teaching is an application of the principle *nemo ad inutile tenetur.* Often, even though medical science has technically perfected a treatment or surgical procedure, the hope of success and benefit does not outweigh the risk involved. Hence, even though there is hope of benefit, it is not a hope of sufficient proportion to make a procedure obligatory. In an article reprinted in the *Linacre Quarterly* in November 1955, Raber Taylor speaks of risks involved in some modern treatments.[19] He relates the case of a man who has a swollen hand. The case was diagnosed as Dupuytren's contracture, and the doctor recommended corrective surgery without, however, disclosing to the patient the considerable risk involved. The operation was unsuccessful. Taylor says, "The operation was skillfully performed, but failed to achieve the expected result. The patient was left with greater disability than he had originally."[20] The author relates this incident in order to note that the doctor in question was legally prosecuted in the civil courts for his failure to disclose properly to the patient the risk involved in the recommended surgery before obtaining the patient's consent. Furthermore, he writes, "The skillful

---

[19] R. Taylor, "Consent for Treatment," *Linacre Quarterly* 22.4 (November 1955): 131–135, reprinted from *The Rocky Mountain Medical Journal,* May 1955.

[20] Ibid., p. 133.

performance of the operation did not, ruled the Supreme Court, excuse the doctor who had breached his duty to make a full disclosure of the surgical risk."[21]

What is of interest in this case is the fact that even the civil laws recognize the element of danger and risk in many modern medical techniques. Hence they protect the patient's right to know the risk before any consent is given. How much more important it is, therefore, for moralists to take cognizance of the possible risk or danger involved in a means of conserving life prior to imposing it as an obligatory ordinary means. If a procedure, whether medical or not, does not offer proportionate hope of success and benefit in the conservation of one's life, it is hardly an ordinary means.

Another point to understand clearly is the fact that in determining whether a means offers proportionate hope of success and benefit, one must consider some relative factors. It is hardly possible to establish categorically that a particular means of conserving life will always offer proportionate benefit under all circumstances and to all people. In other words, it is difficult to establish an absolute norm when determining the required hope of success and benefit in any procedure designed to conserve life. In point of fact, it is difficult to apply an absolute norm to any of the elements of ordinary means. Therefore, it is well to call attention to that fact here.

It does seem that an absolute norm can be established regarding clearly extraordinary means. Certainly, there are means of conserving life that are not binding morally to anyone. We have already referred to Healy's suggestion that two thousand dollars is an amount that no one, even a rich man, is bound to expend for the sake of conserving his life.[22] It would be difficult to dispute the fact that an absolute

---

[21] Ibid.

[22] Healy, *Moral Guidance*, p. 162.

norm exists in regard to extraordinary means, and we shall see this more closely in the discussion of moral impossibility in the next section of this chapter. Suffice it to say now that since an extraordinary means is one that exceeds the strength of men in general, any means that exceeds the strength of men in general is obviously not binding on any man and therefore is an extraordinary means absolutely speaking.

The question of an absolute norm in regard to ordinary means, however, is more intricate. It does not seem that one can successfully establish such a norm, because even the older moralists teach that such a purely ordinary and common means of conserving life as food admits of relative inconvenience and difficulty.[23] Furthermore, they point out that this very common means, food, sometimes can offer no proportionate hope of success relative to a particular individual.

There are many factors in this notion of relativity. For example, the age of an individual can be a determining factor. The person's physical and psychological condition enters the question. His financial status also can weigh heavily in determining a means as ordinary or extraordinary for him. This doctrine on the relative nature of ordinary means should be kept in mind, therefore, in regard to all the elements involved in ordinary means, not only in regard to the hope of proportionate success and benefit.

There is one last point in this connection which is worthy of mention. We have stated that it seems difficult to establish the presence of an absolute norm in regard to ordinary means. We are not denying thereby that there are many means of conserving life which are certainly common means or remedies and which usually do not exceed the

---

[23] See, for example, Vitoria, *De temperantia*, n. 1; and de Lugo, *De justitia et jure*, disp. X, sect. I, n. 30.

strength of men in general. It would be allowable, therefore, to make a *general* norm in regard to these means, by which they are characterized as ordinary for most men. To make this norm absolute, however, it is to imply that these means are obligatory for all men because ordinary means are obligatory means. It is in this sense that we say that it seems difficult to establish a norm which would be absolute in determining the nature of ordinary means.

An application of the relative norm can be made in reference to the element of proportionate hope of success and benefit. Kelly gives the example of the use of oxygen in tiding a patient over a pneumonia crisis.[24] The oxygen is easy to obtain and easy to use and generally is quite inexpensive for short periods of use. If the patient overcomes the pneumonia crisis, he usually will recover from his illness. Kelly writes, "I would say that under these conditions the patient is obliged to use the oxygen if there is any solid hope of getting through the crisis."[25] He then remarks that any change in either the cost or the use of the oxygen which would make its use more difficult would also affect the need for an increase in hope of recovery as a basis for obligation.[26]

There is therefore a definite relation between the notion of proportionate hope of benefit and the nature of ordinary means. The more a means involves difficulty, the more definite must be the hope of proportionate success and benefit. Kelly suggests this principle, and it seems quite valid: "A remedy which includes rather great difficulty, though not moral impossibility, is hardly obligatory unless the hope of success is more probable, whereas a remedy which is easily obtained and used seems obligatory as long as it offers any

---

[24] Kelly, "The Duty of Using Artificial Means," p. 214.
[25] Ibid.
[26] Ibid.

solid probability of success."[27] This seems to be a precise interpretation of the notion of proportionate hope of success and benefit.

In summary, therefore, we may say that the notion of proportionate hope of success and benefit is an essential part of the nature of ordinary means. Without this hope of benefit, a means is hardly an ordinary means and is therefore not obligatory. In determining the presence of this hope of success and benefit, one must consider not only the nature of the particular remedy or means involved, but also the relative condition of the person who is to use this means. Then, and then only, can the moral obligation of using such a means be properly determined.

Means in Common Use
(Media communia)

The next element that is frequently mentioned in referring to ordinary means of conserving life is the notion of being *common*. We have seen this in the writings of Vitoria: "Foods which men commonly use and in the quantity which customarily suffices for the conservation of strength."[28] Sayrus also refers to the need of employing only the means in common use.[29] We note the same in the writings of Sánchez.[30] In a similar manner, de Lugo writes that a man would be guilty

---

[27] Ibid., pp. 214–215.

[28] "Alimentis, quibus homines communiter utuntur et in quantitate quae solet sufficere ad valetudinem conservandam." Vitoria, *De temperantia*, n. 12. See also Vitoria, *Commentarios a la secundae*, q. 147, art. 1.

[29] Sayrus, *Clavis regia casuum conscientae*, lib. VII, cap. IX, n. 28.

[30] Sánchez, *Consilia seu opuscula moralia*, tom. II, lib. V, cap. I, dub. 33.

of suicide not only if he were to kill himself with a sword, but also if he did not conserve his life by common means.[31]

Although the moralists use many expressions to describe the nature of ordinary means, the notion of being common seems to be basic. Even when the expression "common" is not used, it is presumed, and from the whole context, the reader is aware of the presumption. For the moralists, the duty of conserving one's life does not demand a diligence or a solicitude that exceeds the usual care that most men normally give their lives. Any means of conserving life that is not the normal or usual course of action adopted by men in general is out of the ordinary—extraordinary—and therefore *per se* not obligatory. Recall Vander Heeren's phrase that an individual is only bound "to make use of all the ordinary means which are indicated in the usual course of things."[32]

Common diligence therefore, requires the use of common means only. The ordinary conservation of one's life does not imply the singular assiduity involved in prolonging life by unusual and uncommon means. In determining whether or not a means is common, however, it is necessary, of course, to consider the relative factors involved. For this reason, the moralists frequently mention in their writings the next element of ordinary means, namely, one's status in life.

In Keeping with One's Status
(*Secundam proportionem status*)

The element of comparison with one's social position or particular status in life is frequently mentioned by the moralists not only in connection with the notion of common

---

[31] "Non solum dicitur se interimere homo, quando ferro se occidit, sed etiam quando mediis communibus vitam non conservat." De Lugo, *De justitia et jure*, disp. X, sect. I, n. 27.

[32] Vander Heeren, "Suicide," p. 327.

means but also with the notion of the cost involved in using a certain means of conserving life. De Lugo calls attention to it relative to common means.[33] Bañez mentions it in connection with cost.[34] Very often however, the notion of one's status is introduced into the very concept of ordinary means. Reiffenstuel, for example, uses such a method.[35]

De Lugo's example of the comparison with one's status is very interesting and helps to accentuate the principle involved.[36] He notes that Vitoria had taught long before that one who cares for his life by means which other men commonly use certainly is satisfying the obligation of caring for his life. De Lugo then applies this same principle to the religious novice who is advised to return to the world in order to obtain food and surroundings which are more healthful for him. The supposition is that ordinary life in religion is having an ill effect on the novice's life and health. De Lugo prefers to ignore the fact that the novice can licitly be given permission to return to the world. That fact is obvious for de Lugo, but beside the point. The question is whether the novice has the *obligation to return* to the world in order to conserve his life. In other words, must the religious novice who is in ill health exchange the ordinary life of religion for the ordinary life of the world in order to conserve his health? Does the duty of self-conservation require that such a novice relinquish the life men commonly live in the monastery for the life that men commonly live in the world? Is the accent, therefore, only on the expression "common," or must consideration also be given to the particular status that a man has in life?

---

[33] De Lugo, *De justitia et jure*, disp. X, sect. I, n. 36.

[34] Bañez, *Scholastica commentaria*, in II-II, q. 65, art. 1.

[35] Reiffenstuel, *Theologia moralis*, tract. IX, distinc. III, quaes. II, n. 14.

[36] De Lugo, *De justitia et jure*, disp. X, sect. I, n. 36..

De Lugo replies that the obligation of conserving one's life and health does not require the novice to return to the world. He indicates that the novice satisfies his obligation by using food and means which *other men in religion* commonly use to conserve their lives.[37] As a matter of fact, further on de Lugo completely denies any moral obligation in this regard which binds the novice to leave the monastery.[38]

We have cited this case to emphasize de Lugo's teaching that very often one must take into consideration an individual's particular status before a means can be properly determined as ordinary for him. Furthermore, this principle does not apply only to the determination of ordinary means in general; each element of ordinary means must be considered in the light of one's conditions or status. The elements of extraordinary means also are subject to a comparison with one's status in life, and this must be kept in mind too.

It may appear that this element of comparison with one's status is merely the relative norm that we mentioned earlier. The notion of comparison with one's status is contained in that relative norm. Our treatment of it here, however, is no mere repetition of what we have already said. When the authors refer to a comparison with one's status, they seem to be implying a relation with one's social or financial condition. Hence they speak in terms of means being common or ordinary with respect to one's status. They also mention that a means must not be too costly in consideration of an individual's position. The relative norm, however, which we discussed before, is broader than that. It considers not only the financial or social position of an individual but also his

---

[37] "Cur ergo novitius ... nec satisfaciet utendo victu, et mediis quibus alii communiter in religione utuntur et vitam conservant?" Ibid.

[38] "Propter haec itaque existimavi, medicorum illud consilium de obligatione novitii rejiciendum omnino esse." Ibid.

physical condition. The relative norm clearly encompasses also the psychological outlook that an individual possesses in regard to the use of a particular means of conserving life. Our task here has been to discuss the elements which the moralists mention in the light of the discussions which they give. That is the reason that we have allotted separate treatment to the element of comparison with one's status.

Not Too Difficult
(*Non difficilia*)

Many of the moralists show a very definite preference for describing in a negative way the ordinary means of conserving life. They seem to reason that if the elements which make a means extraordinary can be shown to be lacking in a certain means, then the means is clearly an ordinary means of conserving life. Since the difficulty involved in an extraordinary means is usually easier to describe, they seem content to show what an extraordinary means is, and then say that an ordinary means is one which does not entail such difficulty. Hence we note that very often in their writings they use the phrase *media non difficilia.*

Not all authors refrain from a positive expression in this regard. Soto notes that a "prelate could indeed force a subject, on account of a singular obedience promised to him, to take medicines which he can conveniently accept."[39] Sayrus too remarks that "by the natural law each one is bound to employ for the conservation of his body those licit means which he can conveniently undertake."[40]

---

[39] "Prelatus vero cogere posset subditum propter singularem obdientiam illi promissam, ut medicamina admittat quae commode recipere potest." Soto, *De justitia et jure*, lib. V, quaes. II, art. 5.

[40] "Jure naturali media licita, quae commode sumi possunt ad sui corporis conservationem ponere tenetur." Sayrus, *Clavis regia*, lib. VIII, cap. IX, n. 38.

More often, however, the authors prefer to say that one is bound to employ only the means which are not too difficult. For example, Lessius teaches that a man is held to care for his health by ordinary means "which are not extremely difficult."[41] Bonacina uses practically the same words.[42] Laymann also excludes means which are very difficult.[43]

Does any amount of difficulty at all cause a means to be extraordinary? Is it essential to the nature of an ordinary means that the means be entirely free of difficulty? From a study of the writings of the moral theologians, one cannot help but realize that these authors certainly require an *excessive* difficulty before terming a means extraordinary. They clearly state, however, that a *moderate* difficulty does not constitute an extraordinary means. Furthermore, from a study of their writings, one cannot say that the moralists teach that the terms "difficulty" and "ordinary means" are mutually exclusive.

In order to make their teaching clearer, the moralists usually give examples of the elements which they are discussing. When the notion of excessive difficulty is treated, very often the authors use the example of an amputation. These authors consider an amputation an example of excessive difficulty which all will recognize and appreciate. We shall mention the example of an amputation again when we treat the nature of extraordinary means. Here, however, it is worthwhile to call attention to the teaching of Roncaglia in regard to amputation. Roncaglia mentions an amputation as an extraordinary

---

[41] "Mediis ordinariis non admodum difficilibus." Lessius, *De justitia et jure*, lib. II, cap. IX, dub. 14, n. 96.

[42] "Remediis ordinariis non valde difficilibus." Bonacina, *Moralis theologica*, tom. II, disp. II, quaest. ultim., sect. I, punct. 6, n. 2.

[43] "Non tenetur per medium valde difficile." Laymann, *Theologica moralis*, lib. III, tract. III, p. 3, cap. I, n. 4.

means because of the tremendous pain involved. But he also remarks that whenever "from the amputation, future pains of notable proportion will not arise but only moderate pains, then one is bound to suffer the abscission; for everyone is held to conserve his life by ordinary means, and it is an ordinary means to suffer something to conserve this same life."[44]

Roncaglia's phrasing is very clear. It is an ordinary means to suffer moderate pain for the conservation of one's life. Hence we can say that, for Roncaglia, if a means of conserving life involves only moderate difficulty, it is an ordinary means.

Even in the time of Tournely this fact was recognized. Tournely teaches that the proper care of one's life and health can involve difficulty which is only moderate and not excessive.[45] He therefore holds that an individual has the duty of undergoing moderate pain in order to conserve his life. Furthermore, if the individual concerned refuses to suffer such pain, he can be forced to submit to it for the conservation of his life.[46]

The difficulty connected with employing a particular means of conserving life can arise not only from pain, but also from many other elements such as cost, danger to life, fear, etc. The notion of difficulty is generic. Therefore, in a solution of a practical case, consideration should be taken of the possible factors which constitute a difficulty.

---

[44] "Ex abscissione non sint futuri dolores ingentes, sed moderati, tunc tenetur pati abscissione; nam unusquisque tenetur mediis ordinariis vitam conservare et medium ordinarium eat aliquid pati pro eadem vita conservanda." Roncaglia, *Theologia moralis*, vol. I, tract. XI, cap. I, q. IV.

[45] See Tournely, *Theologica moralis*, tom. III, Tract. de Decalogo, cap. II, de quinto praec., art. I, conc. 2.

[46] Ibid.

The theologians require that an individual exert definite effort in conserving his life, but they do not demand any endeavor which could not be expected of men in general. Certainly a means whose use, absolutely speaking, entails a difficulty which exceeds the strength of men in general is not an ordinary means. Furthermore, if a means involves great difficulty for a particular individual, even though men in general do not find any great difficulty in its use, it ceases to be ordinary for this individual. In other words, even if the great difficulty is only relative, not absolute, it is still sufficient to render a means extraordinary for a particular individual. We have mentioned earlier in this chapter that Vitoria applied the relative norm even to food, a very common means of conserving life. It will be profitable now, however, to note the words with which he describes this relative difficulty. Vitoria writes, "If the depression of spirit is so low and there is present such consternation of spirit in the appetitive power that only with the greatest of effort and as though by means of a certain torture can the sick man take food, right away that is reckoned a certain impossibility and therefore he is excused."[47]

The dictate of the natural law that requires a man to conserve his own life is a serious one. It is based on the double importance of man's human life. His life is important, first, as a divine gift over which God retains the ultimate dominion. Secondly, it is important as the means whereby man can merit his eternal salvation. Hence, self-conservation is no mere heroic act which, although laudable, is not obligatory. The conservation of one's own life is not just a desirable

---

[47] "Quod si animi dejectio tanta est et appetitivae virtutis tanta consternation, ut non nisi per summum laborem et quast cruciatum quendam aegrotus possit sumere cibum, jam reputatur quaedam impossibilitas et ideo excusatur." Vitoria, *De temperantia*, n. 1.

thing which entails no serious duty. In reality, the natural law imposes self-conservation as a very definite obligation from which the individual is excused only when such conservation is impossible for him either physically or morally.

The natural law therefore requires that definite effort be expended in the conservation of one's life, even if this involves difficulty. The difficulty, however, must be proportionate. If self-conservation involves excessive difficulty or proportionately grave inconvenience, then certainly the individual is excused. The reason is that the obligation of conserving one's life is a positive precept and as such does not bind with such grave inconvenience and difficulty. We have explained this in chapter 1.

St. Thomas refers to law as an "ordinatio rationis"—an ordinance of reason.[48] A law, to be a true law, commands only what is within reason. Furthermore, the fulfillment of a law need be accomplished only in a reasonable way. Hence, while it is true that one is excused from fulfilling a positive precept when this fulfillment involves grave inconvenience or moral impossibility, he is not excused when he can fulfill it reasonably. Therefore, it is not beyond the bounds of moral obligation to suffer reasonable difficulty in the use of the means of conserving life.

In determining whether a means is reasonable or not, many factors must be considered. One must take into consideration the means contemplated, the objective difficulty involved, and one's own ability to make use of the means. But one must also weigh the importance of the dictate of the natural law which requires one's self-conservation. Any decisions to be made in this matter should be products of a consideration of both the gravity of the law and the difficulty involved in the fulfillment of the law. To ignore the gravity

---

[48] *Summa theologiae* I-II, q. 90, art. 4.

of the law prepares the way for neglect of duty. To ignore the difficulty involved in fulfilling the law fosters scrupulosity.

In our discussions of the element of moral impossibility which we shall treat in the section concerning the nature of extraordinary means, we will refer to the element of difficulty again. The main point to emphasize here, however, is that the nature of ordinary means does not exclude the concept of reasonable difficulty. Hence we say that an ordinary means is one that an individual can reasonably employ in the conservation of his own life.

Reasonably Simple Means
(*Facilia*)

The reader can see in the table on pages 118 and 119 that it was not a common practice of the moralists to include the notion of *easiness* in their discussions of the ordinary means of conserving life. Patuzzi,[49] Waffelaert,[50] and Noldin and Schmitt[51] do mention it. However, in context, the writings of these authors indicate that they did not intend to require a complete lack of difficulty before calling a means ordinary. Rather, they appear to say that ordinary means must be means that one can employ conveniently—in other words, reasonably.

To say that an ordinary means must be easy to use is an expression that can be open to misunderstanding. One might easily imagine that the concept of ordinary means must of necessity exclude any type of difficulty. In the light of the discussion given in the previous section, however, it would seem correct to say that the proper expression is

---

[49] Patuzzi, *Ethica Christiana*, tom. III, tract. V, pars V, cap. X, consec. 7.

[50] Waffelaert, *De justitia*, n. 40.

[51] Noldin-Schmitt, *Summa theologiae moralis*, II, p. 308.

reasonable, not *easy.* Ordinary means are reasonable means. They are not necessarily easy means, because they can entail moderate difficulty.

THE NATURE OF EXTRAORDINARY MEANS

In this section, we shall discuss the elements which are included in the concept of the extraordinary means of conserving life. As in the previous section, we have gathered these elements from the writings of the moral theologians concerning the means of conserving life. Very often these writers used more than one phrase in referring to a particular element of extraordinary means. In the table presented earlier in this chapter, we have included the majority of those phrases. In our treatment of them here in this section, however, it will be more precise to join the elements into five groups in order to focus on the inconvenience involved in the elements rather than on the expression used to describe the inconvenience. Therefore, we shall discuss the elements in the following order: (1) something impossible (*quaedam impossibilitas*), (2) great effort or excessive hardship [*summus labor* and *media nimis dura*], (3) excruciating or excessive pain [*quidam cruciatus* or *ingens dolor*], (4) extraordinary expense and the very best means [*sumptus extraordinarius, media pretiosa,* and *media exquisita*], and (5) intense fear or repugnance [*vehemus horror*].

A Certain Impossibility
(*Quaedam impossibilitas*)

The moral theologians are quite conscious of the distinction between avoiding evil and doing good. They understand clearly that a man is always bound to avoid evil, but he is not always bound to do positive good. There is a limit to the duty of doing good. To the theologians this is a distinction of major importance. Hence, when the theologians discuss the problem of conserving life, they apply the

139

distinction between avoiding evil and doing good to this problem. A man is always bound to avoid suicide because it is intrinsically evil. However, there is a limit to his obligation of conserving his life in a positive manner. The obligation of conserving one's life in a positive way certainly does not include using any possible means, but rather would seem to extend itself to the use of reasonable or moderate means. Hence the theologians apply the term "ordinary" to those means which are reasonable and the term "extraordinary" to those means which a man is not obliged to use in conserving his life. The reason that the extraordinary means are not obligatory is the fact that there is a *certain impossibility* connected with either obtaining or using them. Hence the individual is excused from employing such means.

We have seen clearly in chapter 2 of this dissertation that the excusing cause of impossibility can be licitly applied in regard to the precept of the natural law which binds a person to conserve his life. When an individual is unable to fulfill the law, he is not bound to fulfill it. This inability can be of a physical nature. If, for example, the means of conserving life are certainly unattainable or the individual is physically not fit to make use of these means, he is excused from conserving his life on the grounds of physical impossibility. On the other hand, the individual may be physically capable of fulfilling the law but unable to, here and now, because of some circumstance of fear, danger, or grave inconvenience which renders the observance of the law extremely difficult for him. It is then said to be morally impossible for him to fulfill the law. Hence, if the means of conserving life are excessively difficult or gravely inconvenient to obtain or use, then the use of these means is morally impossible.

It is obvious that physical impossibility excuses from the precept which obliges a man to conserve his life. Everyone understands that no one is bound to use a thing which he can neither obtain nor use. *Nemo ad impossibile tenetur.*

However, in connection with the term "moral impossibility," it is necessary to recall that theologians distinguish the negative and affirmative precepts of the natural law. Negative precepts, such as the prohibition of suicide, are always binding because they forbid something that is intrinsically evil. The application of the excusing cause of moral impossibility therefore is illicit. It is only in regard to the affirmative precepts of the natural law that one can use the excusing cause of moral impossibility.

Self-conservation is an affirmative precept of the natural law and as such binds *semper* but not *pro semper.* When, therefore, a means of self-conservation involves a proportionately grave inconvenience, it is not obligatory, and the individual is excused from the present observance of the precept.

In their discussions of the means of conserving life, the moralists use the terms "certain type of impossibility," "moral impossibility," and "grave inconvenience." For example, Vitoria[52] and Sayrus[53] employ the term "a certain type of impossibility." Mazzotta uses the same expression.[54] On the other hand, Tournely[55] and more recently Marc and Gestermann,[56] Aertnys and Damen,[57] and Kelly[58] make use of the term "moral impossibility." Finally, the term "grave

---

[52] Vitoria, *De temperantia*, n. 1.

[53] Sayrus, *Clavis regia*, lib. VII, cap. IX, n. 31.

[54] Mazzotta, *Theologia moralis*, tom. I, tract. II, disp. II, quaest. I, cap. I.

[55] Tournely, *Theologica moralis*, tom. III, Tract. de Decalogo, cap. II, de quinto praec., art. I, conc. 2.

[56] Marc-Gestermann, *Institutiones morales*, p. 491.

[57] Aertnys-Damen, *Theologiae moralis*, I, p. 566.

[58] Kelly, "The Duty of Using Artificial Means," p. 206.

inconvenience" is used, for example, by Lehmkuhl,[59] Kelly,[60] and Paquin.[61]

We know from the accepted axiom that an affirmative precept is not binding in the presence of a proportionately grave inconvenience. Whether the terms "proportionately grave inconvenience" and "moral impossibility" are synonymous is perhaps open to dispute. Most authors define moral impossibility as a proportionately grave inconvenience which excuses from the present observance of the law. For example, Lucius Rodrigo, S.J., defines moral impossibility as a "proportionately grave inconvenience extrinsic to the observance of a law, but accompanying that observance."[62] Dominicus Prümmer, O.P., says that moral impossibility is present when the prescribed undertaking cannot be accomplished except through very extraordinary effort.[63] Zalba refers to the "inconvenience … which implies great difficulty and lack of proportion in relation to the law concerning which there is question."[64] Lehmkuhl writes that an affirmative law does not bind in the presence of inconvenience but notes that the gravity of the law will determine the required gravity of the inconvenience.[65]

---

[59] Lehmkuhl, *Theologia moralis*, p. 344.

[60] Kelly, *Medico-Moral Problems*, V, pp. 8–9.

[61] Paquin, *Morale et medicine*, p. 344.

[62] "Incommodum proportionate grave et legis observationi extrinsecum, eidem observationi adnexum." L. Rodrigo, *Praelectiones theologico-morales comillenses* (Santander: Sal Terrae, 1944), series I, *Theologia moralis fundamentalis*, II, n. 430.

[63] "Quando opus praescriptum fieri nequit, nisi adhibendo labores prosus extraordinarios." D. Prümmer, *Manuale theologiae moralis* (Freiburg: Herder, 1933), I, n. 235.

[64] "Incommodum … quod magnam difficultatem et improportionem implicat relate ad legem de qua est questio." Regatillo-Zalba, *Theologiae moralis*, I, n. 555.

[65] Lehmkuhl, *Theologia moralis*, I, p. 108.

The authors, when writing in regard to the extraordinary means of conserving life, seem to use interchangeably the terms "moral impossibility" and "proportionately grave inconvenience." It is difficult to determine whether or not they consider them equivalent terms, or whether the expression "proportionately grave inconvenience" implies a difficulty of less magnitude than "moral impossibility." Whatever term they use, the fact remains that these authors insist that the difficulty involved in using a means of conserving life must be of sufficient proportion to constitute an excusing cause before the means can be called extraordinary. It would seem allowable, therefore, to use the terms interchangeably when referring to extraordinary means. Kelly, writing in *Theological Studies,* says that "an extraordinary means is one which prudent men would consider at least morally impossible with reference to the duty of preserving one's life."[66] In *Medico-Moral Problems* the same author writes, "If the inconvenience involved in preserving life was excessive ... then this particular means of preserving life was called *extraordinary.*"[67] Therefore, it is in keeping with the tradition of theological writing in this matter to say that an extraordinary means is a means which is morally impossible because it involves a grave inconvenience not in proportion to the gravity of the precept demanding self-conservation.

We have referred to the words of St. Thomas in regard to law: "ordinatio rationis." Merkelbach, commenting on these words, notes that the term *ordinatio* signifies "dispositio ad finem per media proportionata."[68] He further explains that *rationis* means that the "will of the superior, in order that there can be a law, must be regulated by reason or in

---

[66] Kelly, "The Duty of Using Artificial Means," p. 204.

[67] Kelly, *Medico-Moral Problems*, V, p. 9.

[68] Merkelbach, *Summa theologiae moralis*, I, n. 222.

conformity with reason, otherwise wickedness would result rather than law."[69]

A true law is in conformity with reason, and the means employed to fulfill the law must be in conformity with reason. Since the dictate of the natural law which commands a man to conserve his life is obviously a reasonable law, the means employed to fulfill it need only be within reason. Hence any inconvenience or difficulty that is unreasonable is not obligatory. We may ask how great must be the difficulty or inconvenience involved in self-conservation in order to be unreasonable. Merkelbach says, "How great a difficulty is required to be an excuse must be judged from the importance of the law, the quality of the persons and circumstances of places and times, etc."[70]

The inconvenience involved in using a particular means of conserving life is not just reasonable difficulty. It must be an inconvenience extrinsic to the observance of the law and of sufficient magnitude to be out of proportion to the gravity of the law. A means of conserving life that involves only moderate difficulty and inconvenience is certainly not an extraordinary means. When one has to decide whether or not a means is extraordinary by reason of proportionately grave inconvenience, one must consider both the gravity of the law and the factors involved in establishing the inconvenience. Noldin and Schmitt say that the question of which means are extraordinary must be decided from the common estimation of men.[71] Father Kelly phrases it best of all: "In concrete cases

---

[69] "Voluntas superioris, ut lex esse possit, debet esse ratione regulate sue rationi conformis, secus esset magnis iniquitas quam lex." Ibid.

[70] "Quanta autem difficultas requiratur ut excuset, moraliter aestimandum est ex legis momento, personarum qualitate, circumstantiis locorum, temporum, etc." Ibid., n. 377.

[71] Noldin-Schmitt, *Summa theologiae moralis*, II, p. 308.

it is not always easy to determine when a given procedure is an *extraordinary* means. It is not computed according to a mathematical formula, but according to the reasonable judgment of prudent and conscientious men."[72]

One further point in this matter of moral impossibility concerns the relative norm. Are means to be considered extraordinary only if they involve moral impossibility for men, absolutely speaking, or will relative moral impossibility suffice? A means of conserving life which involves relative moral impossibility must be considered extraordinary. This would be true even if the cause of moral impossibility were unfounded—for example, irrational fear. Kelly writes, "My general impression is that there is common agreement that a relative estimate *suffices*. In other words, if any individual would experience the inconvenience sufficient to constitute a moral impossibility in the use of any means, that means would be extraordinary for him."[73]

We have seen in this discussion that an essential element of extraordinary means is moral impossibility. An extraordinary means of conserving life is one which is morally impossible due to some grave inconvenience out of proportion with the gravity of the law. The elements which we shall discuss in the following sections are actually the possible causes of moral impossibility in a particular means of conserving life. The elements will not always be present in a given means of conserving life. If they are present and render a means extraordinary, it is because they have been the cause of moral impossibility.

---

[72] Kelly, *Medico-Moral Problems*, V, p. 11.
[73] Kelly, "The Duty of Using Artificial Means," p. 206.

Great Effort or Excessive Hardship
(*Summus labor* or *Media nimis dura*)

In our discussion of the moral teaching concerning the ordinary and extraordinary means of conserving life, we have noticed that the natural law requires a man to expend definite effort in order to conserve his life. Any effort which constitutes a moral impossibility, however, is an extraordinary means. Hence, the moralists use such expressions as "the greatest of effort" or "too difficult" when they are describing an extraordinary means.

Tamburini notes that a man is not held to make use of extraordinary foods when this requires tremendous effort, because "love of one's self does not demand such effort."[74]

Patuzzi recalls that Franzoja would oblige a man to employ means which are harsh and difficult and which would require great effort to use. Patuzzi says that this reply came from Franzoja because of Aristotle's teaching that a brave and strong man does not flee difficulty. However, Patuzzi is quick to note that Aristotle is speaking of those who commit suicide in order to flee difficulty and trouble, not about "those who refuse to avoid death at the cost of harsh and severe remedies."[75] He adds then further on that "an individual does not violate the natural law when for a good end and just cause he refuses to conserve his life by extraordinary, rather harsh and violent remedies."[76]

---

[74] "Quia cum tanto labore, nequaquam propria charitas obstrigit." Tamburini, *Explicatio decalogi*.

[75] "Non vero de illis qui vitare mortem recusant mediis acerbis et aerumnosis." Patuzzi, *Ethica Christiana*, tom. III, tract. V, pars V, cap. X, consec. 7.

[76] "Non ergo legem naturae et caritis violabit qui recto fine justaque de causa remediss extraordinariis, acerbioribus, et violentis vitam conservare recusarent." Ibid.

A means which requires excessive effort therefore involves a moral impossibility; thus, it is an extraordinary means. There are many factors in conserving one's life which could cause this effort. In the writings of the earlier moralists, one of the examples of a non-obligatory effort is the example of a long journey to a more healthful land.[77] Many of the authors repeat this example. However, a modern example is given by Zalba. He notes that a man is not bound "to submit himself to a very dangerous operation or to a very burdensome convalescence."[78] Many modern medical and surgical remedies do not give any moral assurance of proportionate benefit. Thus they are extraordinary means. Even where the technique involved in these procedures has been perfected so that they give definite hope of proportionate benefit, however, the very harsh or very troublesome convalescence which follows such procedures could render the remedy itself an extraordinary means. Any means of conserving life which involves the excessive expenditure of effort on the part of the individual concerned is an extraordinary means. Here again the relative norm suffices. If the means involves effort which constitutes a grave inconvenience for the individual concerned, even though most men would find the means reasonable, the means is nevertheless an extraordinary means for this individual.

---

[77] See, for example, Sayrus, *Clavis regia*, lib. VII, cap. IX, n. 28. Paquin, however, says, "Mais cet exemple, dans notre monde moderne, ne peut-etre déjà plus une valeur absolue." *Morale et medicine*, p. 400.

[78] "Neque operandi valde periculosae vel convalescentiae molestissimae se submittere." Regatillo-Zalba, *Theologiae moralis*, II, p. 269.

Excruciating or Excessive Pain
(*Quidam cruciatus* and *Ingens dolor*)

One can readily understand that the element of pain can render a means of conserving life extraordinary. Very often pain is involved in the remedies employed to cure sickness or disease. This is true with modern medical procedures, but it was even more true before the days of anesthesia. Hence we note that pain is almost universally mentioned by the moralists as an element which can cause a means to be extraordinary. The pain involved in a particular remedy can constitute a moral impossibility, and therefore the remedy is an extraordinary means of conserving life, even if the hope of benefit is certain.

The older moralists were very conscious of this fact. They all mention the element of pain. The common example which they give to emphasize this point is amputation. Whenever they write concerning extraordinary means, invariably they mention pain, and almost in the same line cite the example of an amputation. This is not without reason. These authors were writing in the days before anesthesia, when the pain involved in an amputation must have been excruciating. The abscission was painful enough, but this was followed by cauterizing with hot irons to stop the bleeding. For example, the German surgeon Wilhelm of Fabry (1560–1624) is said to have used "a red hot knife for amputation in order to check bleeding!"[79]

Besides the fact that amputation without anesthesia is so obvious an example of intense pain, perhaps the older moralists cited this example so often because in those days amputation was the remedy for almost all compound fractures. The following lines from Douglas Guthrie's *History*

---

[79] Guthrie, *History of Medicine*, p. 150.

of Medicine will help in understanding the conditions of surgical procedures at that time and also why the example of amputation is so constant in the writings of the moralists:

> These were the days in which hospital gangrene assumed epidemic proportions, and sepsis was an inevitable sequence of operations. Compound fractures were treated by amputation, with a mortality of at least twenty-five percent, while the surgeon wore an old blood-stained coat with a bunch of silk ligatures threaded through one of the buttonholes, ready for use. ... Small wonder, then, that a considerable degree of heroism was demanded from the unfortunate patient who, having endured the tortures of operation without anaesthesia, was still obliged to face the pains and dangers of a septic wound.[80]

Science has progressed since the days when there was no remedy for pain. In the Providence of God, the discovery of anesthesia eventually came and brought with it an entirely new outlook in regard to surgical interventions. Contemporaneously, the great scientist Joseph Lister (1827–1912) discovered "the principle involving the prevention and cure of sepsis in wounds."[81] In the course of years, as the antiseptic system was adopted in surgical procedure, the great danger of infection in operations was also almost eliminated; hence, surgical procedures in general today are not as painful or as dangerous as they were in former times. Therefore, many of the procedures which were extraordinary means may be ordinary means now. Consideration must certainly be given to each individual case, however, before a means is determined to be ordinary or extraordinary. It is true that pain is removed during operations by anesthesia, and it is somewhat

---

[80] Ibid., p. 307.
[81] Ibid., p. 324.

lessened in convalescence by sedatives. However, pain and discomfort are still involved in many procedures, and if these elements constitute a proportionately grave inconvenience, then the means is an extraordinary means

Anesthesia has lessened the influence of pain as a factor in causing a means to be an extraordinary means, but it has not eliminated the necessity of considering this element when judging whether or not a means is ordinary or extraordinary.

Furthermore, we must keep the relative norm in mind. The same pain that does not render a means extraordinary for one individual could render it extraordinary for another individual. Hence, prudent judgment above all is necessary.

One must consider not only the pain involved in any surgical intervention—which these days can usually be eliminated—but also the post-operative pain, which usually can be lessened if not eliminated. In this regard, however, the words of Capellmann are significant:

> Although the cure of wounds effected by an operation will bring post-operative pain, this pain is usually not more intense, and is most often less intense, than the pain which the sickness which has caused the operation brings and which the patient would have to suffer even if he did not submit to the operation.[82]

It is well, therefore, to remember that the element of pain must definitely be considered when determining whether a means is ordinary or extraordinary. The effect of anesthesia should be considered. The operative and post-operative

---

[82] "Quamvis deinde curatio vulnerum operatione effectorum postea dolores afferat, hic tamen generatim non atrociores, pleurumque minus sunt atroces, quam illi quod morbus ipse, quo operatio necessaria fiebat, excitavit, quosque aegrotus etiam sine operatione perferre debuit." Capellmann, *Medicina pastoralis*, p. 26.

pain should be considered. The pain in relation to the individual concerned should be considered. If the pain involved would not exceed the strength of men in general and does not constitute excessive inconvenience for this particular individual, the procedure is an ordinary means. Otherwise, it is an extraordinary means.

One further point in this regard refers to an opinion found in the Ballerini-Palmieri edition of Gury's *Compendium theologiae moralis.* The opinion suggests that one would not be bound to accept an artificial means of inducing sleep "as long as such inducing of sleep is a dangerous thing ... because ... certainly it is an extraordinary means: really, the very loss for some time of the use of reason and of the mastery of his acts, such as occurs in this hypothesis, seems an extraordinary thing." [83] One must readily admit that any excessive danger involved in the use of anesthesia in a particular case would certainly render a procedure an extraordinary means. We have already treated this point when speaking of proportionate benefit. However, it does not seem that one could establish that the use of anesthesia is always an extraordinary means on account of the loss of the use of reason and mastery of one's acts. We have stated that the inconvenience involved in a procedure must be out of proportion with the gravity of the law. Since we are discussing at this time a means which is to be employed for the conservation of one's life, it does not seem that the inconvenience involved in the temporary loss of the use of reason would be out of proportion to the duty of self-conservation. Anesthesia is hardly an extraordinary means on that account. A case is possible, though, in which a person would have an excessive fear of losing the use of

---

[83] Gury-Ballerini-Palmieri, *Compendium theologiae moralis,* n. 391; the Latin text is given above in chapter 2, note 117.

reason. Then the means might become extraordinary, not because of the loss of the use of reason but because of the excessive fear. We shall discuss this element of fear in another section of this chapter.

Extraordinary Expense and the Very Best Means
(*Sumptus extraordinarius, Media pretiosa,* and *Media exquisita*)

The moral theologians have always taken into account the element of expense when discussing the ordinary and extraordinary means of conserving life. They have constantly taught that any means of conserving life which imposes an excessive hardship on an individual because of cost is an extraordinary means. In other words, unreasonable expense can constitute a moral impossibility and thus render a means extraordinary. To describe this excessive cost involved in conserving one's life, the moralists use such general terms as *sumptus extraordinarius, media pretiosa,* and *media exquisita.*[84] We have noted earlier in this chapter that the authors speak very frequently of the relative norm in regard to expense. It is apparent from their writings that any expense which causes a grave inconvenience for a particular individual renders a means of conserving life an extraordinary means. We have noted also in this chapter that when the moralists speak of cost, they frequently use the expression *secundum proportionem status.* Hence, the relative norm in this matter suffices.

It is not the practice of these authors, even the recent ones, to establish a definite expense beyond which an individual is no longer obliged.[85] However, there is nothing in their

---

[84] Bañez, however, writes that three thousand ducats is an extraordinary means. See *Decisiones de iure et iustitia,* in II-II, q. 65, art. 1.

[85] See Healy, *Moral Guidance,* p. 162.

writings which is opposed to establishing an absolute norm. In fact, if anything, their writings favor an absolute norm.[86] But one will not find the practice of stipulating a definite amount as an example of expense which is an extraordinary means, absolutely speaking. The theologians are, no doubt, mindful that monetary values change and that the income of individuals changes. Furthermore, the amount of money that constitutes a moral impossibility, absolutely speaking, for people of one country might easily be reasonable for people of another country. Hence the authors leave the determination of absolute expense in the matter of extraordinary means to the contemporary and native moralists.

The history of the problem of the ordinary and extraordinary means of conserving life shows that expense has always been considered an essential factor in determining a means ordinary or extraordinary. This is no less true these days. The progress of science has brought about substantial improvements in medical procedures and technique. The cure of ills and the conservation of life has been greatly advanced. However, the question of expense is still a very real problem and, in reality, is perhaps an even greater problem than before. R. Cunningham, writing about an American private health insurance plan, says,

> The constantly growing complexity of medicine has made medical care increasingly expensive. Diagnosis today is far more exact than it was even twenty years ago, but it often requires many expensive laboratory tests. And many modern treatments also are

---

[86] For example, Joseph Sullivan says, "On the other hand, no one, not even a very wealthy person is obliged, *per se*, to call in a very expensive physician. ... There is an absolute norm beyond which means are *per se* extraordinary." *Catholic Teaching on the Morality of Euthanasia* (Washington, D.C.: University of America Press, 1949), p. 64.

costly. ... Other studies have shown that one fifth of the nation's families are in debt for hospital or medical bills, and that medical care commonly takes from 4 to 7 per cent of family income and, in a few cases, as much as 40 per cent.[87]

The cost of medical and surgical treatments which require hospitalization vary. Some treatments are not too expensive. For example, one hospital estimates $1330 as the cost of hospitalization for a case of acute appendicitis with no complications.[88] The price includes the cost of the operating room, anesthesia, medication, and hospital ward accommodations for eight days. On the other hand, the cost of hospitalization for diabetes mellitus involving a gangrenous ulcer of the right foot and a low tibial amputation is estimated at $892.10.[89] The ward accommodations in this case are for sixty-one days. The price is broken down in the following way:

Operating room	$17.50
Anesthesia	30.00
Laboratory	257.50
Medication	154.10
Medical & surgical supplies	6.00
Board: 61 days at $7.00 a day	427.00
Total	$892.10[90]

---

[87] R. Cunningham, *The Story of Blue Shield* (New York: Public Affairs Committee, 1954), p. 2.

[88] St. Joseph's Hospital, Reading, Pennsylvania. The cost sheet was prepared by Sister M. Fridoline, O.S.F., and submitted to me for use in this dissertation.

[89] Ibid.

[90] EDITOR'S NOTE: A note here in 1988 edition of this work reads, "Hospital charges today are based on diagnostic related groups (or DRGs). Through the kindness of John W. Logue, President of

The reader will note that in both cases the cost is only for hospitalization and does not include the fees of either the doctor or the surgeon.

We can see, therefore, that expense is involved even now in the conservation of one's life. However, there are additional factors in the question of cost that must be considered. First, public hospitals exist, and very often the cost of medical treatment, at least the full cost, does not have to be paid by the patient.[91] Secondly, some countries, such as England, have a health service whereby medical treatment is paid for from public funds. Thirdly, there are private insurance plans, as for instance in the United States. With such insurance, a patient is greatly aided in meeting medical bills which would otherwise be impossible for him to pay. We can understand, therefore, that medical expense must be considered in the light of the individual's financial condition.

The tradition of moral teaching in regard to the means of conserving life shows that consideration must be given to the question of expense. The cost involved will render the means an extraordinary means if it is excessive for the individual concerned. Here again, however, prudent judgment must be used in making the decision, and consideration must

---

Carney Hospital, Boston, Massachusetts, the following figures have been made available for comparative purposes. According to the database presently in effect at Carney Hospital, the average charge for an appendectomy without complications (DRG 167) would be $3,050 (average length of stay, 3.7 days). For any operation on the cranium for an individual under age 17—no trauma (DRG 001)—the average charge would be $24,874 (average length of stay, 36 days)." Charges today would clearly be much higher.

[91] See Ubach, *Theologia moralis*, I, n. 488, where he notes that extraordinary cost is often absent because a surgical operation is usually performed in a public hospital.

be given not only to the expense but also to the gravity of the duty of self-conservation.

Intense Fear or Repugnance
(*Vehemens horror*)

The final element which the moralists consider in their discussions of extraordinary means is *vehemens horror*. There are two main emotions to which the authors give attention. One is intense fear. The other is very strong repugnance.

The emotion of fear helps a man to protect his life. It is because of fear that a man withdraws from what is harmful or injurious. Fear causes a man to escape from danger. Yet "fear is sometimes so intense that it paralyzes the subject and leaves him unable to move."[92] Fear, being a natural emotion, quite obviously is present when certain means of conserving life come into question. When an individual considers the pain or other inconveniences involved in a particular procedure, fear can cause him to shun this means of conserving life. In certain cases, the fear of a particular procedure can be so intense that it constitutes a moral impossibility. Thus the procedure becomes an extraordinary means. There are medical procedures which can cause fear, even excessive fear, in most men. However, in any practical decision, one must consider the emotional or psychological condition of the individual concerned. If the fear is excessive and causes a grave inconvenience, the means in question is an extraordinary means.

Sometimes this excessive fear may be unfounded. It may be unwarranted by the objective danger or pain involved in a procedure. In this case, the individual concerned should rid himself of this unnecessary excessive fear. He should

---

[92] T. Gannon, *Psychology: The Unity of Human Behavior* (Boston: Ginn and Company, 1954), p. 254.

consider the matter objectively. Fear that is irrational should be eliminated, if possible, before determining whether or not a means is extraordinary. However, if the excessive fear remains, irrational and unwarranted though it be, the means can constitute an extraordinary means. Thus, the fear provides a legitimate excuse from employing such a means of conserving life.[93]

Repugnance, or distaste for a particular means, is also mentioned by the moralists in their writings. Usually in this connection they give the example of a maiden who is unwilling to submit to any medical treatment by a male doctor, when this is repugnant to her sense of modesty.[94] This resolve on the part of the maiden, whereby she prefers the pains of illness, even death itself, to the inconvenience caused by repugnance to treatment by a male doctor, is perhaps unwarranted. The fact remains, nonetheless, that this intense distaste can constitute a moral impossibility. Patuzzi does not agree. He calls this repugnance imprudent and inane. Furthermore, this author says that the maiden ought to subject her emotions to the law of charity and the law of nature.[95] However, it seems that most moralists would agree that if the maiden's repugnance causes a moral impossibility, then the treatment by a male doctor is for her an extraordinary means.

One final point in this section concerns another example in regard to the element of repugnance. We have mentioned before that the moralists cite an amputation as an example

---

[93] See Ubach, *Theologia moralis*, I, n. 488.

[94] See, for example, Busenbaum and St. Alphonsus, n. 372; the Latin text is given above in chapter 2, note 81.

[95] See Patuzzi, *Ethica Christiana*, tom. III, tract. V, pars V, cap. X, consect. sept.; the Latin text is given above in chapter 2, note 111.

of an extraordinary means, owing to the grave danger and intense pain involved. Science has improved the technique in operations, and thus an amputation is no longer as dangerous as it was. Anesthesia has removed the pain. Yet repugnance to living with a mutilated body could just as readily constitute a grave inconvenience. This point also should be remembered when determining whether such a procedure is an ordinary or extraordinary means for a particular individual.[96]

We can see, therefore, that these two factors, fear and repugnance, must be considered when judging whether a procedure is an ordinary or extraordinary means of conserving life. The relative norm is of particular importance in regard to this element. A procedure which causes no fear or repugnance at all for men in general might easily be a source of grave fear or intense repugnance for a particular individual. If, therefore, the fear or repugnance constitutes a moral impossibility, it renders the procedure an extraordinary means of conserving life.

SUMMARY OF MORAL OBLIGATIONS

We have studied up till now the writings of the moral theologians in regard to the ordinary and extraordinary means of conserving life. We have noticed that no set definition of these terms has been given, but that the authors simply described these means. From the descriptions and the examples given by these writers, we have been able to gather the essential elements involved in the terms "ordinary and extraordinary means." We have collected the elements that are constantly used and have studied what is implied in these elements. Hence, we actually have the essential

---

[96] See Ballerini-Palmieri, *Opus theologicum*, II, p. 645, n. 868, note b; the Latin text is given above in chapter 2, note 118.

concepts which the tradition in moral writings requires for ordinary and extraordinary means.

Definitions of
"Ordinary" and "Extraordinary"

Gerald Kelly is one of the very few moralists to attempt a definition of these terms. He restricts the definition, however, to hospital procedures. He writes, "As regards hospital procedures, *ordinary means* of preserving life are all medicines, treatments, and operations which offer a reasonable hope of benefit for the patient and which can be obtained and used without excessive expense, pain or other inconvenience."[97] In reference to *extraordinary means*, he says, "By these we mean all medicines, treatments, and operations, which cannot be obtained or used without excessive expense, pain or other inconvenience, or which, if used would not offer a reasonable hope of benefit."[98] Hospital procedures are not the only means of conserving life. Hence, a definition of ordinary and extraordinary means must be broad enough to include any means which is used for conserving life. Furthermore, an ordinary means is one which excludes the notion of moral impossibility, but it does not exclude the notion of reasonable difficulty.

The elements to be included in the nature of ordinary means, as we have noted, are definite hope of proportionate benefit, the notion of being common, and reasonable effort. In contrast, extraordinary means involve the notion of lack of proportionate benefit and the notion of moral impossibility arising from unreasonable inconvenience in regard to pain, fear, expense, or such.

---

[97] Kelly, *Medico-Moral Problems*, V, p. 6.
[98] Ibid.

Since all these elements have been shown to be constant in the moral teachings concerning the ordinary and extraordinary means of conserving life, we suggest the following definitions:

> *Ordinary means* of conserving life are those means commonly used in given circumstances, which this individual in his present physical, psychological, and economic condition can reasonably employ with definite hope of proportionate benefit.

> *Extraordinary means* of conserving life are those means not commonly used in given circumstances, or those means in common use which this individual in his present physical, psychological, and economic condition cannot reasonably employ or, if he can, will not give him definite hope of proportionate benefit.

The reader will notice that these definitions are based on the relative norm. In this matter the relative norm suffices for judging whether a means is ordinary or extraordinary. However, if there is a question of absolute grave inconvenience, then the same definition of extraordinary means is obviously valid. In regard to ordinary means, we have previously eliminated the use of an absolute norm.

Thus far in this chapter, we have been discussing the nature of the ordinary and extraordinary means of conserving life. We now intend to discuss the obligation of using these means. The usual manner of phrasing this obligations in: *per se* a man is obliged to use the ordinary means of conserving his life; *per se* he is not obliged to use extraordinary means, though the use of extraordinary means might be obligatory *per accidens*.[99]

---

[99] See Kelly, "The Duty of Using Artificial Means," p. 206.

Obligation to Use Ordinary Means

Zalba emphasizes the gravity of the obligation to employ the ordinary means to conserve one's life.[100] Our life is a precious gift of God, and it provides an essential condition in this economy by which we can merit heaven. Hence the care of our life is a serious obligation and imposes the duty of employing the ordinary means necessary for such care. Not to employ the ordinary means of conserving life is tantamount to suicide and is thus a grave sin. One who refuses to employ the ordinary means of conserving his life equivalently kills himself.[101]

We have included the notion of utility or proportionate hope of success and benefit as an essential part of our definition of ordinary means. Any means, therefore, that does not give definite hope of benefit is an extraordinary means. This element has been shown to be included constantly by the moralists in the concept of ordinary means. Sometimes, however, confusion on this point can occur. Some authors speak of ordinary means and hope of benefit as two separate entities. Then they join the two notions in order to determine the obligation of using the ordinary means. The implication is that one can determine a means as ordinary apart from the notion of proportionate benefit.

Kelly writes, for example, "The patient is *per se* obliged to use only those means which are ordinary and which offer a reasonable hope of success."[102] Discussing a practical case concerning a particular means of conserving life he says, "But

---

[100] "Cura vitae conservandae et administrandae imponit obligationem, ex genere suo gravem, positive procurandi et applicandi media congrua." Regatillo-Zalba, *Theologiae moralis*, II, p. 298.

[101] See Genicot-Salsmans, *Institutiones*, I, p. 298.

[102] Kelly, "The Duty of Using Artificial Means," p. 216.

even granted that it is ordinary, one may not immediately conclude that it is obligatory."[103] Kelly is actually carefully noting that all attendant circumstances must be weighed before a means of conserving life can be called ordinary and obligatory.

In order to avoid this confusion, we have based our definition on the relative norm. Thus, if a means of conserving life is ordinary in accordance with our definition, it is automatically obligatory. It is precisely because of this possible confusion that we have stated that an absolute norm for ordinary means cannot be admitted. Since the obligation of conserving life rests with the individual primarily, it would seem that the ordinary means should be determined in accordance with the conditions of the individual. Once the means are then determined as ordinary means for this individual, they are obligatory

Again it is well to read that this method is in no way opposed to establishing a *general norm* whereby means are characterized as ordinary for most men. But in the last analysis, the individual's own conditions will determine a means as ordinary or extraordinary. That is the reason we have based our definition on the relative norm; it is also the reason why we can say that ordinary means of conserving life are always obligatory.

Obligation to Use Extraordinary Means

All authors admit that reasonable care of one's life does not include the use of extraordinary means. Hence *per se* extraordinary means are not obligatory. The moralists, how-

---

[103] Ibid., p. 218. In later writings, Kelly includes the notion of usefulness in his definitions of ordinary and extraordinary means; see his definitions in *Medico-Moral Problems* above (at notes 96 and 97) and in "The Duty to Preserve Life," p. 550.

ever, do note that extrinsic circumstances can change a case. They admit that for some reason a person might be bound to take more than ordinary care of his life, particularly when there is question of prolonging one's life. For this reason, they say that an individual might be bound *per accidens* to employ even extraordinary means of conserving his life.[104]

The usual examples of those who are obligated *per accidens* to use extraordinary means are (1) one who is especially necessary to his family or society[105] and (2) one who should prolong his life for his spiritual welfare.[106]

For example, suppose that the father of a large family is dangerously ill. The doctors give him moral assurance that by means of a surgical intervention he can regain his health. However, the post-operative pain will be very intense and for him will constitute a moral impossibility. In this case the means of conserving life is considered extraordinary. Hence, the individual has *per se* no obligation to use this means to conserve his life. However, the extrinsic circumstance of a large family could change the case. The means of conserving life is still extraordinary; his duty of his own life still does not demand the use of extraordinary means. But his duty to his family could oblige him to make use of a means which he would not otherwise be bound to employ. Hence, in such a situation, the individual is said to have the obligation *per accidens* of using an extraordinary means of conserving his life.

In regard to the second example, we may cite this case. A patient is dying in great pain. Death is certain and inevitable. He is a Catholic but has been away from the Sacraments for twenty years. He is willing to see a priest

---

[104] See Regatillo-Zalba, *Theologiae moralis*, II, pp. 268–269.
[105] Ibid.
[106] Kelly, "The Duty of Using Artificial Means," p. 206.

and receive the Sacraments. A certain drug may prolong his life for another hour or two. Must he take the drug in order to stay alive long enough to receive the Sacraments?[107] Our reply is as follows. The drug in question is an extraordinary means because the physical benefit to be derived from its use is negligible. Death is certain. There is no proportionate hope of benefit. Since the drug, therefore, is an extraordinary means, it is not obligatory *per se*. However, the patient has the grave obligation of making his peace with God and receiving the Last Sacraments. Thus, the hour or so that will be given him by using the drug are necessary for him in order to see a priest. From the obligation, therefore, of caring for his soul, the obligation arises *per accidens* of prolonging his life by using an extraordinary means. Hence, in this case the patient is bound *per accidens* to use the drug in question.

The principle involved in this matter is very clear, namely, extraordinary means are obligatory only *per accidens*. Applications of this principle can be complicated, however, because the circumstances of a case can be involved. Prudent judgment above all is necessary. It must be remembered that the common tendency of most men is to conserve their lives by any possible means. However, their moral obligation extends *per se* only to the use of the ordinary means, and only *per accidens* to the extraordinary means.

In this chapter, we have seen the nature of the ordinary and extraordinary means of conserving life. We have seen that the relative norm suffices in determining a means as ordinary or extraordinary. We have also mentioned that there can be an absolute norm in regard to extraordinary means according to which certain means are not obligatory for any

---

[107] This case is a modification of one presented for discussion by Charles McFadden, O.S.A. See C. McFadden, *Medical Ethics* (Philadelphia: F. A. Davis, 1955), p. 159, case 11.

man *per se*. Furthermore, we stated that a *general norm* can be established whereby certain means are classed as ordinary means for most men, although we emphasized that in the last analysis only the relative norm will determine an ordinary means. Finally, we reviewed the principles involved in the obligation to use the means of conserving life. We noted that means which are ordinary according to our definition are obligatory means. Extraordinary means are not obligatory except *per accidens*.

Chapter 4

PRACTICAL CONSIDERATIONS

RISK IN MODERN MEDICAL AND SURGICAL PROCEDURES

In the previous chapter, we discussed the nature of the ordinary and extraordinary means of conserving life. In that discussion, we noted that one of the factors which must be considered in determining a means as ordinary or extraordinary is the notion of hope of success. This factor is very important, especially in the determination of modern surgical operations as ordinary or extraordinary means of conserving life. Certainly surgical interventions involve risk. This was true particularly in past ages, but it is also true today. Modern operating technique, with the advances and progress of medical science, has greatly reduced the risk of death, but it has not eliminated risk of death completely.

Traditionally, the moralists have listed amputations and incisions into the abdomen as constant examples of extraordinary means. Published rates of success in such operations today are not sufficiently broad in scope to enable the moralist to render a categoric opinion about the moral problem of "element of risk" in these operations. However, it is interesting to note by way of illustration that in sixty-three recorded cases of leg amputations, five deaths are reported; in 2,454 recorded cases of appendectomy operations, eight deaths are recorded, and finally in 1,382 reported cesarean sections, three deaths are reported.[1]

The indications of the reported causes of death are that complications extrinsic to the operating technique, as well as the physical condition and age of the patient, have been generally the factors responsible for death in the cases cited here. In the report submitted by St. Joseph's Hospital, Reading, Pennsylvania, there is this important observation: the individual patient must be considered with particular emphasis on old age. Mortality, for example, listed under hip surgery more often is caused by age rather than the surgery. Surgery is more the occasion than the efficient cause.[2]

---

[1] These figures appear in lists of operations obtained from the following hospitals: Lynn Hospital, Lynn, Massachusetts; St. Joseph's Hospital, Reading, Pennsylvania; St. John's Hospital, St. Louis, Missouri; St. Mary's Hospital, Decatur, Illinois; St. Elizabeth's Hospital, Belleville, Illinois; and Sacred Heart Hospital, Eau Claire, Wisconsin. For their generous cooperation in preparing these figures and giving permission for the use of them, I am indebted to the authorities of these hospitals. I have made use also of the following article: C. Sullivan and E. Campbell, "One Thousand Cesarean Sections in the Modern Era of Obstetrics," *Linacre Quarterly,* November 1955, pp. 117–126. In this article, the authors present a study of one thousand consecutive cesarean sections performed by the staff of St. Elizabeth's Hospital, Brighton, Massachusetts. The authors report that "in this series of 1,000 consecutive sections, 3 mothers died, a mortality of 0.3%. ... None of the 3 deaths was in any way associated with the technic of cesarean section, and all were emergency procedures" (p. 123).

[2] Report prepared by James Diamond, M.D., and R. Impink, M.D., of St. Joseph's Hospital, Reading, Pennsylvania, and submitted to me for use in this dissertation.

Another observation from this report mentions that operating techniques have not changed too radically. Lowering of mortality rates is due more to connected issues. Above all other such issues the one factor most responsible is the science of anesthesia which has greatly advanced in the past 15 years. It is common practice now to have an MD specialist in anesthesia rather than a nurse as formerly. With this set-up the operating surgeon has a freer mind and hand. Other connected issues are intravenous feedings, blood transfusions (plasma and direct); also antibiotics which greatly reduce danger of infection. Pre-operative checks especially for the aged also reduce mortality: electrocardiographs, chest x-rays, blood chemistry.[3]

The element of risk has been greatly reduced because of modern advances. However, every surgical operation contains a certain amount of risk, and this should be considered in any classification of surgical procedures as ordinary or extraordinary means.

The discussion of the element of risk in surgical operations leads directly to the consideration of modern medical and surgical treatments as ordinary or extraordinary means of conserving life.[4] The reader will recall that we noted in

---

[3] Ibid.

[4] EDITOR'S NOTE (2011): The editors of the 1989 edition of this work placed a footnote here stating that the address to an International Congress of Anesthesiologists by Pope Pius XII (November 24, 1957) appeared "to validate, in general, the discussion in this section ... with regard to the obligation to 'use only ordinary means.'" The editors also drew attention to the more recent "Declaration on Euthanasia" (1980) from the Congregation for the Doctrine of the Faith: "It is also permissible to make do with the normal means that medicine can offer. Therefore

chapter 3 that there is no *absolute norm* for designating a means of conserving life as an *ordinary means*. This is true because of the many relative factors involved in the medical treatment of each individual patient. However, we did admit that one could classify certain procedures as ordinary means according to a *general norm*. In other words, there are some medical treatments which usually are ordinary means of conserving life for men in general, even though certain relative considerations may render them extraordinary means for particular individuals.

Many of the older moralists considered surgical operations extraordinary means because of the pain, expense, and risk of death involved. We have mentioned in the previous chapters that anesthesia has lessened the effect of the element of pain, and that expense also has been diminished because of public hospitals and insurance plans. However, these factors must be considered, because there is still an element of danger in the use of anesthesia and because post-operative pain and inconvenience can constitute even now a moral impossibility. Furthermore, the inconveinence of expense has by no means been removed completely; expense can still constitute a moral impossibility.

The element of risk has been lessened also, but it is still present, particularly in operations performed on elderly patients and on those patients who have a relatively weak constitution. It would seem, however, that *as regards the operating technique,* most common operations offer sufficient hope of success *in the case of young patients* to be termed ordinary means of conserving life. For example, a leg amputation, from the aspect of *operating technique,* does not

---

one cannot impose on anyone the obligation to have recourse to a technique which is already in use but which carries a risk or is burdensome" (sect. 4). As in that edition, these two works are included in appendices here.

involve excessive danger for a young patient in the normal case, and hence from that viewpoint the procedure would be an ordinary means. On the other hand, the danger involved in this operation in the case of an elderly patient is much greater, and in most circumstances such a procedure would be an extraordinary means of conserving life.

Furthermore, the circumstances of the operation affect the situation. The risk ordinarily involved in a cesarean section or an appendectomy performed in a modern hospital with all the advantages of skilled surgeons, anesthesia specialists, and antiseptic facilities would not be sufficient to render these procedures extraordinary means on that account. However, the same procedure performed in one's home, in a less modern or a rural clinic, or by a less capable doctor could easily be an extraordinary means owing to the risk involved.

Major surgery of the more radical type still remains today an extraordinary means of conserving life and health because of the danger involved. For example, the various types of neurosurgery are not morally obligatory for the patient.

A practical summary of the classification of modern surgical interventions as *moral* ordinary or extraordinary means, *from the aspect of the operating technique alone,* would be as follows: (1) Common surgery, even though major surgery, performed on patients of relatively young age and relatively strong constitution and in surroundings which offer the advantages of modern hospital skill, precautions, and equipment is *generally* an ordinary means of conserving life. (2) Major surgery, even though common surgery, performed on patients of advanced age or of relatively weak constitution cannot be classed *generally* as an ordinary means of conserving life. (3) Major surgery, even though common surgery, performed on the young or the old in surroundings which do not offer the advantages of modern hospital skill, precautions, and equipment cannot be classed *generally* as an ordinary means of conserving life. (4) Radical surgery which involves great risk and danger, or which is still insufficiently tested, is an extraordinary means of conserving life both for the young and the old.

The above summary is only in regard to the *operating technique,* so that expense, pain, and repugnance can still determine a means as ordinary or extraordinary. It is on the basis of repugnance that leg amputations probably still remain extraordinary means of conserving life for most people even in these days. This certainly is true in the case of the amputation of both legs.

From the viewpoint of medical treatment, we may say that the initial visit to or calling of a doctor and the examination by him[6] are ordinary means in the case of a person who is seriously ill, as is also ordinary nursing care. However, repeated expense in this matter can render the means extraordinary. The basic medicines, intravenous feedings, insulin, the many types of antibiotics, oxygen masks and tents, preventive medicines and vaccines are ordinary means of conserving life. However, even in these treatments, the relative physical, psychological, and economic condition of an individual can change the case. For example, an extreme horror of needles could easily render repeated injections as extraordinary means for a particular individual. Furthermore, the relative benefit to be derived from an intravenous feeding can be slight in an individual case, and thus the intravenous feeding will be an extraordinary means, as we shall see further on in this chapter.

Blood transfusions *in general* are ordinary means of conserving life unless the expense involved renders them extraordinary means or unless the condition of the patient

---

[6] Notice, however, the exception made in the case of the maiden whose sense of modesty would render an examination by a male doctor extremely repugnant, and hence, for her, such an examination could be an extraordinary means.

provides little hope of benefit from the transfusions. An interesting aspect of blood transfusions is discussed by John Ford, S.J., in the *Linacre Quarterly*.[7] The author studies the refusal of blood transfusions by Jehovah's Witnesses. Jehovah's Witnesses believe that such transfusions involve eating blood, which is contrary to the biblical prohibition found in the Old and New Testaments (Lev 3:17 and Acts 15:29); hence they refuse such treatment. The question arises then as to whether a blood transfusion should be considered an ordinary means of conserving life for the Jehovah's Witness. Ford maintains that the mistaken frame of mind which the Jehovah's Witness possesses in this matter makes the blood transfusion for him an extraordinary means of conserving life. He writes,

> With a sincere Jehovah's Witness who is firmly convinced that a transfusion offends God, we are dealing with a case where his conscience absolutely forbids him to allow the procedure. In this mistaken frame of mind, he would actually commit sin if he went against his conscience and took the transfusion. I see no inconsistency in admitting that this frame of mind is a circumstance which makes the transfusion for him an *extraordinary* means of preserving life.[8]

In general, however, blood transfusions are to be considered ordinary means of conserving life, in the theological sense, just as they are certainly an ordinary medical procedure.

---

[7] J. Ford, "The Refusal of Blood Transfusions by Jehovah's Witnesses," *Linacre Quarterly*, February, 1955, pp. 3–10.

[8] Ibid., p. 6. John Connery, S.J., prefers to consider the blood transfusion as an ordinary means for the Jehovah's Witness and excuses such a patient from using it on the basis of invincible ignorance. See his "Notes on Moral Theology," *Theological Studies* 16 (1955), p. 571.

APPLICATION TO THE DOCTOR

Up to now, our study of the ordinary and extraordinary means of conserving life has been limited to a consideration of the duty of *each individual* to conserve his own life. In other words, we have prescinded, thus far, from any discussion of the extension of this duty to those persons who may be charged with the conservation of another's life, such as relatives, physicians and surgeons, and such. In this present section, therefore, we shall consider the duty of employing the means of conserving life as it applies to the doctor. (We are including physicians and surgeons under the term "doctor.")

There are many obligations which are binding on the doctor by reason of his professional calling. These obligations begin even in medical school, where he has the duty of learning the science of medicine.[9] What concerns us here, however, is the doctor's particular duty to heal and cure. We are interested in the *source* of this obligation and the *content* of the obligation.

The doctor is bound, in general, by the law of God and his professional oath to take care of the sick, although *per se* he is free to accept or not accept a particular person as a patient. This obligation to take care of the sick can stem immediately from the *virtue of charity* and the *virtue of justice*.

The Virtue of Charity

The virtue of charity obliges all men to aid their neighbors who are in need. This need may be spiritual or temporal, and both may be extreme, grave, or ordinary. Jone describes the obligation this way:

---

[9] See A. Bonnar, *The Catholic Doctor* (London: Burns Oates and Washbourne, 1952), pp. 157–162, for a discussion of "The Doctor in His Practice."

In extreme spiritual necessity we must assist our neighbor even at the risk of our life. ... In extreme temporal necessity our neighbor must be helped even at our great personal inconvenience, but not at the risk of our life, unless our position or the common welfare demand the safety of the threatened party. ... In grave spiritual or temporal need our neighbor must be helped in as far as this is possible without a serious inconvenience to ourselves. ... In ordinary spiritual or temporal necessity one is not obliged to help his neighbor in each and every case."[10]

The virtue of charity therefore obliges all men to aid their neighbors who are in need. The doctor's obligation from charity to assist the sick is but a simple application of the general demands of the virtue of charity. Hence, a doctor is bound to take care of a sick man who is ill and needs medical attention if no other doctor is nearby who can and will aid this sick individual.[11] The gravity of the obligation depends, naturally enough, on the degree of necessity in which the sick man finds himself. The doctor's obligation, therefore, can be very grave, serious, or slight according to whether the urgency of the sick man's illness is extreme, grave, or ordinary.

Since the duty of charity is a positive obligation, it is not binding in the presence of a proportionately grave inconvenience. "The proportion can be less rigorous when the demands of charity are less strict."[12] Hence, only a very

---

[10] Jone, *Moral Theology*, pp. 85–86, nn. 138–139.

[11] See F. Hürth, *De statibus* (Rome: Pontificia Universitas Gregoriana, 1946), p. 106.

[12] La proportion peut même être ici moins rigoureuse, puisque les exigences de la charité sont moins strictes." Paquin, *Morale et Medicine*, pp. 102–103.

grave inconvenience will excuse a doctor from taking care of a sick man in extreme need; only a grave inconvenience will excuse him if the person is in grave need, and any real inconvenience will be sufficient to excuse him from caring for a person in ordinary need.

Furthermore, besides this obligation of charity to our neighbor in general, we are bound in a special way to help the poor. Jone describes this obligation in the following way:

> In a case of *extreme necessity* one is obliged under grave sin to help the poor even by sacrificing things necessary for our state of life. ... In a case of *grave necessity* one must help the poor if it can be done without sacrificing things necessary for one's state in life. ... In their *ordinary need* one must help the poor in general from one's superfluous possessions.[13]

This obligation obviously enough applies to the doctor too. Hence, the doctor has the very grave duty to assist gratuitously a poor person in extreme need. He also has the grave obligation to assist gratuitously a poor person in grave need, and a slight obligation to help a poor man in ordinary need. In these cases we also suppose that the man in question is the only doctor available who is willing and able to take care of the sick man, and that the doctor can render his services without a proportionately grave inconvenience.

The Virtue of Justice

Besides the obligation which the virtue of charity imposes on the doctor, a duty can also arise from the virtue of justice. The doctor is bound in justice to visit and take care of the sick with whom he has a contract or a quasi-contract.

A contract exists when the services of the doctor are engaged, orally or in writing, for the purpose of caring for

---

[13] Jone, *Moral Theology*, pp. 86–87, n. 141.

a particular person or group of persons.[14] A quasi-contract exists when the doctor responds to the "call" of a sick person and implicitly agrees, on the promise (at least implicit) of payment, to continue his services as long as the condition of the patient requires them.[15] In these instances, the patient has a strict right to the services of the doctor, and the doctor is bound in justice to render the services. A proportionately grave inconvenience, however, can excuse a doctor from his obligation as long as the inconvenience is one which is not inherent in the professional work itself.[16] For example, a doctor's own illness will excuse him, even though his obligation in the matter is one of justice. However, the danger of a contagious disease will not excuse him from caring for a person whom he is obliged in justice to assist.

Since the doctor is bound to take care of the life and health of the sick, he is obliged to employ the means of conserving life. Hence, the next point is in regard to the doctor's obligation to use the ordinary and extraordinary means of conserving life.

The Doctor and Ordinary Means

Certainly, the doctor has the obligation *per se* of using the ordinary means of conserving life when he treats a patient. Otherwise, he would have no obligation at all. If the doctor were not bound to employ the ordinary means, *a fortiori,* neither would he be bound to employ the extraordinary means. Thus, the question would be closed, and no further discussion would be warranted here. The doctor's basic duty is described very well by Francis Connell, C.Ss.R: "The doctor is bound by the law of God, as well as by his

---

[14] See Paquin, *Morale et Medicine*, p. 101.

[15] Ibid.

[16] Ibid., p. 102.

Hippocratic Oath, to preserve the life of a patient as long as is reasonably possible. This means that ordinary measures must be employed even in the case of one who will continue to be, naturally speaking, merely an unprofitable burden on society."[17]

The moralists recognize this obligation of the doctor, although some phrase it in a manner different from Connell's. For example, Genicot and Salsmans write, "The doctor is bound in justice to furnish the safer or better remedy to a sick person."[18] Implicitly contained in this statement is the obligation of using ordinary means. If the doctor is bound to use safer or better remedies, *a fortiori* he is bound to supply the ordinary remedies. There are other moralists, however, who write in a manner similar to Connell's. Charles McFadden, O.S.A., says, for example, "It is never permissible to hasten the death of any product of human conception. The degree of deformity does not change the situation. . . . The *ordinary* steps to conserve life must be taken."[19] Davis writes that doctors sin seriously if they do not use reasonable and ordinary precautions, for their duty is to keep patients alive, and they have no privilege of killing them.[20] Franz Hürth, S.J., notes that "even if a doctor has

---

[17] F. Connell, *Morals in Politics and Professions* (Westminster, MD: Newman Press, 1951), p. 121.

[18] Medicus ex *justitia* tenetur ad *remedium tutius* seu melius aegroto praebendum." Genicot-Salsmans, *Institutiones theologiae moralis*, I, n. 701. Similarly, Vermeersch, *Theologiae moralis principia-responsa-consilia*, II, n. 492; Aertnys-Damen, *Theologiae moralis*, I, n. 1250; Noldin-Schmitt, *Summa theologiae moralis*, II, n. 743–744; Capellmann, *Medicina pastoralis*, p. 35; G. Payen, *Déontologie medicale d'après droit natural, résumé* (Zikawei, China: Imprimerie de la Mission Catholique, 1928), p. 40.

[19] McFadden, *Medical Ethics*, p. 151.

[20] Davis, *Moral and Pastoral Theology*, II, p. 127.

assumed the care of a sick person from charity alone, he is bound in strict justice to ordinary diligence."[21]

In other words, just as the patient himself is bound to accept the ordinary means of conserving life, so also the doctor is bound to employ the ordinary means of conserving life when he is treating his patient. The patient's refusal to furnish the ordinary measures is equivalent to suicide. The doctor's refusal to furnish the ordinary measures is equivalent to murder. That is why in the *Code of Ethical and Religious Directives for Catholic Hospitals*, one reads, "The failure to supply the *ordinary means* of preserving life is equivalent to euthanasia."[22]

We have stated that a proportionately grave reason will excuse the doctor from ministering to a patient. This teaching applies to the use of ordinary means. A proportionately grave inconvenience which is not inherent in the doctor's professional work will excuse him from his obligation in justice to supply the ordinary means of conserving life. (Recall that this applies also to the care of a patient whom the doctor accepts *ex caritate sola,* since the doctor even in this case is bound *in justice* to employ the ordinary means of conserving life.)

The determination of the doctor's obligation to heal and cure is sufficiently clear in the common case in which

---

[21] Etsi vero medicus curam aegroti ex sola caritate assumpsit, tamen ad diligentiam ordinariam tenetur ex justitia stricta." Hürth, *De statibus,* p. 107.

[22] *Code of Ethical and Religious Directives for Catholic Hospitals* (St. Louis: Catholic Hospital Association of the United States and Canada, 1949), p. 5. In the current (1981) Catholic directives, titled *Ethical and Religious Directives for Catholic Health Facilities*—as approved by the National Conference of Catholic Bishops as the national code "subject to the approval of the bishop for use in the diocese," November 1971—the phrase above is found in directive no. 28.

ordinary means is all that is necessary for the patient's recovery. Obviously, the doctor is obliged to employ the ordinary means in such a case. However, the difficulty arises in cases in which a patient's illness requires treatment by extraordinary means and cases of incurable illness or old age. In cases of this type, one may ask whether the doctor is obliged to go beyond the use of ordinary means and also employ extraordinary means to conserve his patient's life and health. Thus we come to the doctor's obligation of using the extraordinary means of conserving life when he is treating a patient.

The Doctor and Extraordinary Means

It might appear at first glance that the doctor's obligation of employing the means of conserving life is coextensive with the patient's obligation of using these means. A deeper investigation of this problem, however, reveals that this opinion is not complete. Kelly writes in this regard,

> It is easy to show that this statement is inaccurate. The patient is *per se* obliged to use only those means which are ordinary and which offer a reasonable hope of success. But he may use other means, and if he reasonably wishes to use them the relatives and physicians are strictly obliged to carry out his with.[23]

The patient and the doctor are bound to use ordinary means. The patient can refuse to use extraordinary means. If, however, the patient chooses to employ the extraordinary means of conserving his life, the doctor has no choice but to follow the patient's wishes. Hence, we can see that in determining the doctor's obligation to employ the extraordinary means, the first step is to ascertain the patient's own desires in this regard. In the last analysis, it is the patient who has the right to say whether or not he intends to use the extraordinary

---

[23] Kelly, "The Duty of Using Artificial Means," p. 216.

means of conserving life. Therefore, the patient's refusal to accept the extraordinary means immediately releases the doctor from any obligation of employing these means. However, when the patient desires the use of extraordinary means, the situation is different.

Before we attempt to determine the doctor's obligation when the patient desires the use of extraordinary means, it will be helpful to have the following distinctions in mind. (1) *The patient accepted ex caritate and the patient to whom the doctor is bound ex justitia to assist.* This distinction has been sufficiently explained earlier in this chapter. (2) *The expressed request of the patient (explicit or implicit) and his unknown desire.* The patient can expressly request the use of extraordinary means, either explicitly himself or through others, or implicitly by his general attitude in regard to caring for his health. Perhaps, however, his desire of using or not using extraordinary means is entirely unknown. For example, he may be unconscious or delirious. (3) *Absolute extraordinary means and relative extraordinary means.* The absolute extraordinary means are considered morally impossible for all men. The relative extraordinary means are those means which are extraordinary either for the patient alone or for the patient and doctor both. (4) *Useful extraordinary means and useless extraordinary means.* The former give definite hope of proportionate success and benefit, whereas the latter do not.

Case 1

The first possibility is the case which involves a patient *ex caritate*, who needs extraordinary means to conserve his life. He asks the doctor to employ these means. In this case, if the extraordinary means are absolute extraordinary means, the doctor is not bound to employ them in order to conserve the life of the patient. There is no obligation in charity to do for others what one is not obliged to do to save his own life.[24] If the extraordinary means is extraordinary relative only to the patient (for example, an operation that is extraordinary by reason of the extreme pain that it causes the patient) and will be of benefit to the patient, then the doctor is bound to employ such a means. The reason is that charity demands that one assist his neighbor in extreme need even at the cost of serious inconvenience to one's self. However, if this means of conserving life is useless or if it will be of benefit to the patient but will cause a proportionately grave inconvenience to the doctor, then the doctor is not obliged to supply the means. The doctor need not supply a useless means, because no one is bound to use what is useless. The doctor is excused in the second case because we are not bound in charity to employ extraordinary measures to help our neighbor when this is a source of proportionately grave inconvenience to us. This is true even if the means will be of benefit to our neighbor.

The particular obligation of charity to the poor can present an even more specialized problem for the doctor. Imagine the case of a poor man for whom a necessary medical treatment is an extraordinary means by reason of the expense involved. The poor man requests the treatment. In this case, if the doctor can supply the treatment without a proportionately grave inconvenience to himself, he is obliged to supply it. However, a proportionately grave personal inconvenience would excuse him from his obligation. Hence, "a surgeon need not perform an extraordinary operation gratis."[25]

Case 2

The second possibility involves the patient *ex caritate* who needs an extraordinary means to conserve his life. His

---

[24] Jone, *Moral Theology*, p. 87, n. 141.
[25] Ibid.

desires, even implicit, however, in regard to the use of the extraordinary means are unknown. Is the doctor bound to use these extraordinary means?

If the means will not be of benefit to the patient, the doctor's obligation extends only to the use of ordinary means, and he need not employ the extraordinary means. However, if the means would be of proportionate benefit to the patient, the doctor should make a reasonable attempt to determine whether or not the patient would desire the use of extraordinary means. After this investigation, if the doctor believes that the patient would want the extraordinary means, then the doctor should follow the norms given in case 1. If, however, it is entirely unknown what the patient himself would want, and this cannot be determined, then the doctor's duty of charity does not bind him to employ the extraordinary means, even though such means would be of benefit to the patient. We are not bound in charity to force a neighbor to save his life by means which he personally is not bound to use to save his own life. A doctor who would use extraordinary means to save a person's life when the doctor has not ascertained the patient's own wishes would be in effect forcing the patient to use means which the patient himself is not morally obligated to use.

Case 3

The third possibility involves the patient *ex justitia* who reasonably wishes the use of an extraordinary means to conserve his life. In this case, the doctor is strictly obliged to carry out the patient's wish. We may phrase the obligation of the doctor in the case of a patient *ex justitia* this way: "The doctor is obliged to supply those means which the patient is bound to use and reasonably wants to use."[26]

---

[26] See Paquin, *Morale et Medicine*, p. 402.

Case 4

The fourth possibility involves the patient *ex justitia* who needs an extraordinary means to conserve his life. It is unknown, however, whether or not he wishes to use this extraordinary means.

Since the doctor is unable to ascertain the patient's own wishes in the matter, he should make a reasonable effort to determine what the patient's wishes would be if the patient personally could respond. In the event that relatives are present, they should try to make the decision in the name of the patient, and the doctor is obliged to follow their wishes. If there are present no relatives nor persons entrusted with the patient's welfare, then it is up to the doctor to make the decision. His obligation in justice to the patient binds him to take reasonable care of the patient. He must consider the spiritual, physical, financial, and social condition of the patient. Perhaps the doctor will require the aid of others in making this consideration, but in the last analysis it is the doctor's duty to do what he thinks will bring about the greater good of the patient. If the doctor judges that the use of extraordinary means is not the better course to take, then he should feel free in conscience to follow his judgment.

Quite often it is the doctor alone who really can judge the benefit of using an extraordinary means anyway. Even when the patient is able to make the decision, he is not always capable of it either because of lack of knowledge or because of emotional upset. The relatives and friends may be disturbed; they may lack good judgment; they may shun the responsibility of making the decision. The doctor can be level-headed in a situation where the patient or relatives of the patient may not be. If the patient and relatives rely on the doctor's judgment when they *themselves* are responsible for the decision, then the doctor should make a reasonable judgment and feel free to follow it when *he alone* is responsible. The failure to use extraordinary means when the doctor judges this the better course of action is not euthanasia. The doctor, having considered the aspects of the problem reasonably and conscientiously, should feel that he has satisfied his duty in charity and justice to his patient. He has satisfied also his oath to "use treatment to help the sick according to my ability and judgment."[27]

There are cases in which the doctor does not experience too much difficulty in deciding what he should do. The moral issues are clear. For example, Connell mentions the following case and gives a solution with which moralists and doctors would agree:

> If the child whose physical constitution is so defective that he will grow up to be a driveling idiot is seriously ill with pneumonia, the physician must employ the most effective remedies he knows in order to cure him, provided they can be reckoned as ordinary means. There is no obligation to use extraordinary remedies to preserve a life so hampered. Thus, if this child needed a very difficult and delicate operation, which only a specialist could perform, in order to prolong its life, there would be no obligation on the parents or on the doctor to provide such an operation.[28]

However, the doctor, forced to make a decision personally, can find himself involved in a situation more complicated than the one which Connell describes. In his doctoral dissertation, *Catholic Teaching on the Morality of Euthanasia*, Rev. Joseph Sullivan gives the following case:[29] A patient is

---

[27] See the Hippocratic Oath in McFadden, *Medical Ethics*, p. 456.

[28] Connell, *Morals in Politics and Professions*, p. 121.

[29] Sullivan, *Catholic Teaching on the Morality of Euthanasia*, p. 72.

dying of cancer. He is in extreme pain and drugs no longer offer him any extended relief from the pain because he has developed a toleration of any drug given him. Since the disease is incurable and the patient is slowly dying, the doctor wants to stop the intravenous feeding in order to end the suffering. The doctor believes that otherwise, since the patient has a good heart, he will linger on for several weeks in agony. He therefore stops the intravenous feeding and the patient dies. A similar case is presented by Joseph Donovan, C.M., in the *Homiletic and Pastoral Review.*[30] Neither author specifically mentions whether or not the patient is conscious, or whether or not there are relatives who can make the choice. In his reply, Sullivan says,

> Since the cancer patient is beyond all hope of recovery and suffering extreme pain, intravenous feeding should be considered an extraordinary means of prolonging life. The physician was justified in stopping the intravenous feeding. He should make sure first, however, that the patient is spiritually prepared.[31]

Contrary to this opinion, Donovan writes,

> I fear that to neglect intravenous feedings is a form of mercy killing rather than a means of sustaining life that is morally impossible to use. Here is a cancerous person given three months to live, and he cannot be nourished except by intravenous means, is he therefore to be let starve to death, even if he is willing?[32]

Sullivan has carefully mentioned many conditions in his presentation of the case. It would seem, therefore, that

---

[30] J. Donovan, "Letting Patients Die," *Homiletic and Pastoral Review* 49 (August 1949), p. 904.

[31] Sullivan, *Catholic Teaching on the Morality of Euthanasia.*

[32] Donovan, "Letting Patients Die."

the intravenous feeding is an extraordinary means for the cancerous patient concerned. Even in the situation related by Donovan, it would be licit to consider the intravenous feeding an extraordinary means of conserving life.[33] However, recall that we based our definition of ordinary and extraordinary means on the relative norm. In the presumption, therefore, that a doctor alone has the responsibility to make a decision in a particular case, he should consider all the conditions of the patient, because intravenous feeding cannot be called an ordinary means of conserving life *absolutely speaking*, even though according to a *general norm*, it may be an ordinary means for most men.

---

[33] EDITOR'S NOTE (2011): More recently, specific guidance on questions concerning artificial nutrition and hydration has been provided by the Congregation for the Doctrine of the Faith, as well as by the 2009 edition of the *Ethical and Religious Directives for Catholic Health Care Services* (n. 58). The CDF states that for those in a persistent vegetative state, "the administration of food and water even by artificial means is, in principle, an ordinary and proportionate means of preserving life. It is therefore obligatory to the extent to which, and for as long as, it is shown to accomplish its proper finality, which is the hydration and nourishment of the patient. In this way suffering and death by starvation and dehydration are prevented." The CDF recognizes, however, that "the possibility is not absolutely excluded that, in some rare cases, artificial nourishment and hydration may be excessively burdensome for the patient or may cause significant physical discomfort, for example resulting from complications in the use of the means employed." Congregation for the Doctrine of the Faith, "Responses to Certain Questions of the USCCB concerning Artificial Nutrition and Hydration," August 1, 2007, reprinted in *Ethics & Medics* 32.11 (November 2007): 1. See also United States Conference of Catholic Bishops, *Ethical and Religious Directives for Catholic Health Care Services*, 5th ed. (Washington, DC: USCCB, 2009), directive 58.

If, after due consideration of the particular case before him, the doctor decides that the intravenous feeding is an extraordinary means for the patient concerned, he should then follow the norms we have given above for the doctor's use of extraordinary means in the treatment of patients. Cases of this nature must be solved in individual instances after prudent consideration of the condition of the patient concerned. General norms are guides and helps, not the definitive solutions of each similar case. The doctor must use great prudence, but he must also feel free to follow his considered judgment. Euthanasia is illicit and intrinsically evil. However, when all that the doctor can do to cure the person has been done, prolonging a patient's life by an extraordinary means is not the only morally justifiable alternative. It is licit *per se* to refrain from using an extraordinary means of conserving life.

Even more intricate than the cases just mentioned is the problem presented by Ford in his article on the refusal of blood transfusions by Jehovah's Witnesses. We have seen that Ford rightly judges blood transfusions as extraordinary means for Jehovah's Witnesses. Since blood transfusions are extraordinary means in such cases, they are not obligatory. Ford then makes this application to the doctor's obligation in the matter:

> The consequence of this opinion for the physician is obvious. Where the patient is not morally obliged objectively to make use of a procedure, and actually refuses it, the physician is not morally obliged to give it to him; nor do the hospital administrators have a moral obligation to see that he gets it.[34]

Ford next discusses the doctor's position when faced with the care of a child who needs a transfusion but whose parents are Jehovah's Witnesses. Must the doctor regard the blood

---

[34] "Ford, "The Refusal of Blood Transfusions," p. 7.

transfusion as an extraordinary means for this child, even as he would consider it such for the child's parents? Is it licit for the doctor to refrain from giving the transfusion in such a case? Or must the doctor consider the transfusion as ordinary means, as it is for most men, according to the general norm? Is the doctor therefore bound to give the blood transfusion to the child of Jehovah's Witnesses? Ford replies,

> In this case of a young child, therefore, it would be morally wrong to make an agreement not to administer a transfusion in cases of serious need; and if such an agreement were made, one would have no obligation to honor it. The obligation of physicians and others who have actually undertaken to care for the child would ordinarily be an obligation of justice as well as charity. Others who have not actually undertaken the care of the child might have an obligation of charity to intervene in order to see to it that a neglected child is properly cared for.[35]

Ford adds, however, that many factors must be considered which could render quite difficult the possibility of the doctor's carrying out his obligation in this regard. Hence, this author notes further, "After all, his [the doctor's] legal position is far from clear; and it is no small matter to undertake a surgical procedure on a young child contrary to the express refusal of the parents to allow it."[36]

ADDITIONAL FACTORS

Ford's consideration of the doctor's legal position leads directly to our next point. Up to now, we have been treating of the doctor's obligation merely from the aspect of his duty to his patient in charity or justice or both. We have seen

---

[35] Ibid., p. 8.
[36] Ibid., p. 9.

his obligation of charity to his neighbor in general and to
the poor in particular. We have also seen his obligation in
virtue of the patient–physician contract, namely, a duty in
justice. However, a question arises as to whether or not the
doctor's complete duty in the matter of using the extraordinary means of conserving life is sufficiently explained
merely from his moral obligations of charity and justice in
regard to his patient. Are the moral obligations of charity
and justice to the patient the only obligations that bind a
doctor in this matter?

Kelly, in his writings on medical ethics, has emphasized
on more than one occasion the need to consider the doctor's
professional ideal whenever we discuss the doctor's obligation
of using the extraordinary means of conserving life when
he is treating a patient. Kelly first makes reference to this
point in his article "The Duty of Using Artificial Means of
Preserving Life" when he writes,

> As for the physicians, there may be another, and
> perhaps more important difference. I have spoken
> of this matter occasionally with very conscientious
> physicians, and I have found that they consistently
> express a professional ideal to the effect that they
> must use all means in their power to sustain life,
> and that they must use any remedy which offers any
> hope, even a slight hope, of cure or relief. ... I do not
> know how common this professional ideal is. But
> from my own experience with physicians and from
> many recent statements of the medical profession
> against euthanasia I would conclude that it is very
> common among conscientious physicians.[37]

In a later article in *Theological Studies,* "The Duty to Preserve Life," Kelly writes more at length on the same subject,

---

[37] Kelly, "The Duty of Using Artificial Means of Preserving
Life," pp. 216–217.

namely, the suggestion that the physician's professional ideal may create obligations that extend beyond the duties and wishes of the patient.[38] This last article is reprinted substantially in another article written by the same author in *Medico-Moral Problems*, "The Extraordinary Means of Prolonging Life."[39] The influence of Kelly's writing on theological discussions of this subject cannot be denied. He has emphasized the need for investigating the duty that arises for the doctor from his obligations to the common good and from his professional ideal and standard.

The subject of the doctor's duty to conserve life by extraordinary means was discussed at the 1952 meeting of the Catholic Theological Society of America in Notre Dame, Indiana. Rev. John Goodwine, in the *Proceedings*, reports on the seminar discussion at that time.[40] He notes that it was generally felt by those present that "the physician–patient contract alone is not sufficient to explain the obligation which physicians feel is theirs, viz., to do more than use ordinary life-saving means."[41] This author then notes that "it is extremely difficult to find a definite and clear statement of the duties physicians owe to their profession."[42]

In order to obtain some idea of what possible obligations may be binding on the doctor in virtue of his duty to

---

[38] Kelly, "The Duty to Preserve Life," pp. 550–556. Kelly does not state whether he considers this an obligation in the strict sense or merely a professional preference.

[39] Kelly, *Medico-Moral Problems*, V, pp. 11–15.

[40] J. Goodwine, "The Physician's Duty to Preserve Life by Extraordinary Means," *Proceedings of the Seventh Annual Convention* (Washington, D.C.: Catholic Theological Society, 1952), pp. 125–138.

[41] Ibid., p. 133.

[42] Ibid., p. 134.

the common good and to his profession, Kelly has recourse to the medical profession itself. He has examined the ideals which conscientious doctors themselves enunciate. From his findings, Kelly has been able to group these ideals under two standards. One he calls the "strict professional standard" and the other, the "moderate standard."[43] Doctors in the first group believe that "the doctor's duty is to preserve life as long as he can, by any means at his disposal, and no matter how hopeless the case seems to be."[44] These doctors think that "insofar as the judgment is left to the doctor himself he must simply keep trying to prolong life right to the very end."[45] The moderate standard is embraced by those doctors who

> try to effect a cure as long as there is any reasonable hope of doing so; they try to preserve life as long as the patient himself can reap any tangible benefits from the prolongation. But they also think there is a point when such efforts become futile gestures; and they believe that at this point the sole duty of the doctor is to see that the patient gets good nursing care and that his pain is alleviated.[46]

The strict standard certainly avoids any type of "euthanasia mentality." However, Kelly notes that the moderate standard has many good features: (1) it is consistent with the policy of the theologians by which they place a reasonable limit on obligations, (2) it is in harmony with the "good Christian attitude" toward life and death, and (3) it is less likely to burden the relatives of the patient with excessive strain and expense.[47]

---

[43] Kelly, *Medico-Moral Problems*, V, pp. 12–13
[44] Ibid.
[45] Ibid., p. 13.
[46] Ibid.
[47] Ibid., pp. 13–14.

Since the publication of the above-mentioned articles, a very significant statement has appeared in print. Dr. A. E. Clark-Kennedy delivered the inaugural address at the opening meeting of the 218th Session of the Royal Medical Society of Edinburgh, an address reprinted under the title "Medicine in Relation to Society" in the *British Medical Journal.* In this address, Clark-Kennedy says,

> Now, it is always easier to perform a palliative operation or put the patient on deep x-ray treatment or chemotherapy; easier, in fact, to do something than to do nothing. Some course of action will probably relieve his immediate symptoms, and often it prolongs his life. It will raise hopes and sometimes clear the bed for the admission of another case for whom more might be done. But what happens to the patient in the end? ... The Roman Catholic doctor in dealing with his Roman Catholic patient has firm guidance from his Church in these matters, and some may hold the view that it is always our duty to prolong life so far as is possible, but my experience teaches me that most of the non-Catholic laity would, if they knew the truth, wish doctors to exercise more moral courage than in point of fact is, I think, their practice in these situations. If the patient or his relatives really could be told the facts, they would have their doctor withhold treatment when "the game is up," and let nature take its course. ... It is written, "Thou shalt not kill." But letting nature take its course when nature cannot be stopped is not killing. Nor in my judgment is a patient committing suicide when he refuses palliative or problematical, as opposed to a reasonably certainly curative, medical or surgical treatment. Never before in the history of medicine has it been so important to remember Clough's oft-quoted rider ... "But needst not strive officiously to keep alive." ... If I really thought that I was either under a moral obligation to keep all my patients alive as

> long as possible, or under a legal obligation always
> to apply the textbook treatment for the textbook
> disease, I would give up medicine tomorrow![48]

The statement indicates the vexation that besets the doctor
when he faces the problem of prolonging a patient's life.
Clark-Kennedy betrays a lack of complete understanding of
the Catholic teaching in this matter; the Catholic Church
does not demand that the doctor preserve life as long as
possible.

However, the doctor has very skillfully presented a
legitimate problem, a problem which at times can be very
disturbing to the physician. Science has progressed in the
treatment of some diseases—only far enough, however,
to prolong the patient's life, not cure the disease. Clark-
Kennedy's statement also reveals that evidently there is no
agreement among doctors themselves as to a course of action
which might be called a general rule in this matter.

A similar statement has been made by an American
general practitioner. Dr. Francis Hodges of San Francisco
writes,

> The hopelessly ill patient need not, through a
> distorted sense of professional duty, be subjected
> to heroic and extraordinary measures, whose only
> purpose can be prolongation of an existence that
> has become intolerable. But it must be the patient
> himself who declines the measures.... Let us sense
> those times when we must not reach into the
> bottom of our medicine bags for agents to whip
> into a body tired unto death a final, additionally
> exhausting further fight against death, a death for
> which the patient is already prepared. ... There are
> times when the patient has legal, ethical, moral and

---

[48] A. E. Clark-Kennedy, "Medicine in Relation to Society,"
British Medical Journal, March 12, 1955, pp. 620–621.

religious justification of his request to be allowed
to die in peace.[49]

The medical profession itself realizes the problem, but "as yet
there is no clear-cut professional standard regarding ... the
'fine points' of care of the dying."[50] The medical profession
may very well look to the moralists for the answer, just as Kelly
has consulted doctors in order to attempt an appreciation
of their ideals. However, when this problem of the doctor's
obligation (arising from his duty to his profession and the
common good) of using extraordinary means was discussed
at the seventh meeting of the Catholic Theological Society,
Goodwine reports, "it was generally felt that until more is
known about the doctor's obligation to society, no satisfac-
tory and clear-cut statement of their duty to use extraordinary
means can be drawn up."[51] Kelly notes that "among moral
theologians a somewhat similar condition prevails; up to a certain point duties are clear and there is agreement on what must
be done; beyond that point the rules of obligation become
obscure and there is room for differences of opinion."[52]

Conceivably, the doctor may believe that the advancement of medical science requires him to do all in his power to
prolong life and to attempt a cure even though at the time all
seems hopeless. Confronted with an apparently hopeless case,
the doctor realizes that even the present advances of science
do not enable him to cure his patient. Certainly, ordinary
means will not cure the patient; perhaps even extraordinary
means will not effect a cure. Yet the doctor senses the igno-
miny of giving into death, and he finds himself constrained

---

[49] F. Hodges, quoted in *Time* (Atlantic ed.), January 9,
1956, p. 31.

[50] Kelly, *Medico-Moral Problems*, V, p. 14.

[51] Goodwine, "The Physician's Duty to Preserve Life," p. 138.

[52] Kelly, *Medico-Moral Problems*, V, p. 14.

to fight the disease to the best of his ability, perhaps even by employing insufficiently tested methods and procedures. He realizes that medical knowledge has grown over the years and in great measure this has been due to experience with patients. Hence, the doctor is not content to let his patient refuse the extraordinary means of conserving life. He considers doing so a betrayal of his duty to the furthering of medical science.

Furthermore, the doctor may be confronted with a patient whose life he could almost surely save if the patient would accede to the use of extraordinary means. The doctor believes though that agreement with the patient's wishes is euthanasia and, therefore, contrary to his professional oath and ideal.

Yet the doctor must realize that although the advancement of medical knowledge is good in itself, there are other factors that must be considered. The conquest of medical problems is not the only duty of the doctor. He has the primary duty of *treating the patient* lying before him—that human being weak with illness who wants his help and his services but who perhaps does not want health at the price of using clearly extraordinary measures. The advancement of medicine is a worthy motive, but it is a motive clearly limited, and it can never justify the doctor's forcing a patient to use extraordinary means of conserving his life.

The doctor must use the ordinary means of conserving life. He must also use those extraordinary means which the patient wants to use. He must continually study and attempt to find a remedy to the disease which afflicts his patient, but he must also remember that his prime duty is to his patient, not to his profession. Hence, any extraordinary procedure which the patient refuses, or which the doctor believes the patient would refuse if he were able to understand the problem more competently, is not obligatory for the doctor, because it is not obligatory for the patient, and the advancement of science or the doctor's professional ideal does not change that fact.

The duty to conserve a patient's life rests primarily with the patient himself. Since the patient is not morally obligated to use an extraordinary means, it seems highly unlikely that a doctor's profession can make him force the use of an extraordinary means on a patient. Clearly, too, the non-use of extraordinary means when the patient refuses them is not euthanasia.

This same manner of thinking must guide the doctor in treating a patient who cannot make a decision in regard to the use of extraordinary means and who has no one to make the choice for him. The doctor should judge the case reasonably and decide what will effect the greater good for the patient and then act accordingly. But he should never judge that an unconscious patient, a charity patient, or a mentally ill patient whose life is in extreme danger should be given treatment by extraordinary measures merely for the advancement of scientific and medical knowledge or because he believes his professional ideal requires him to fight death right to the end. The doctor should treat the patient, not just the disease. Euthanasia is illicit, but so also is surreptitious experimentation carried out by the use of extraordinary means of conserving life without the consent of the patient.

The doctor may also believe that the common good requires him to employ extraordinary means of conserving his patient's life. However, the doctor must remember that while it is incumbent on all to work for the common good, in this problem we are dealing with the question of a man's life. The prime responsibility for the conservation of one's life rests with the individual. The individual, *per accidens*, may be peculiarly necessary for the common good and thus be bound to conserve his life even by using extraordinary means. In this case, the doctor would be bound to employ these extraordinary means. However, when the common good does not demand that the patient himself use the extraordinary means of conserving life, it is difficult to see how the doctor can be bound, on account of the common good, to employ extraordinary means when he is treating this same individual.

Jules Paquin writes,

> It is evident that the doctor must avoid the appearance of negative euthanasia, that he ought to avoid giving the impression of letting his patients die. But it is not opposed to the common good that a doctor, in certainly incurable cases, cease costly treatments which have no other effect than to prolong for a while a life, at times, already unconscious.[53]

In practice, therefore, a doctor should take his norm from the obligations of the patient himself. The doctor must employ the ordinary means of conserving life and then those extraordinary means which, *per accidens,* are obligatory for the patient or which the patient wants to use. He must never practice euthanasia, and he must conscientiously strive never to give the impression of using euthanasia. Furthermore, he must strive to find a remedy for the disease. However, when the time comes that he can conserve his patient's life only by extraordinary means, he must consider the patient's wishes, expressed or reasonably interpreted, and abide by them. If the patient is incurable and even ordinary means, according to the *general norm,* have become extraordinary for this patient, again the wishes of the patient expressed or reasonably interpreted must be considered and obeyed. Kelly gives this practical norm:

---

[53] "Il est évident que le médecin doit éviter l'apparence de l'euthanasie négative, qu'il doit éviter de donner l'impression de laisser mourir ses maladies. Mais le bien commun ne s'oppose pas à ce qu'un médecin, dans des cas certainement incurables, cesse des traitements couteux que n'auriaient pas d'autre effet que de prolonger très peu une vie parfois déjà inconsciente." Paquin, *Morale et Médecine*, p. 402.

When a doctor and his consultants have sincerely judged that a patient is incurable, the decision concerning further treatment should be in terms of the patient's own interest and reasonable wishes, expressed or implied. Proper treatment certainly includes the use of all natural means of preserving life (food, drink, etc.), good nursing care, appropriate measures to relieve physical and mental pain, and the opportunity of preparing for death. Since the professional standards of conscientious physicians vary somewhat regarding the use of further means, such as artificial life-sustainers, the doctor should feel free in conscience to use or not use these things, according to the circumstances of each case. In general, it may be said that he has no moral obligation to use them unless they offer the hope of some real benefit to his patient without imposing a disproportionate inconvenience on others, or unless, by reason of special conditions, failure to use such means would reflect unfavorably on his profession.[54]

The common good and a doctor's professional ideal do oblige him to keep trying to find a remedy for disease. What we have said about the doctor's obligation to follow the wishes of the patient is, therefore, not to be interpreted as a hindrance to further medical knowledge. Hence, a doctor should not interpret this teaching as being opposed to the trial of new medical procedures or cures. Within certain limits, it is licit to attempt a cure with extraordinary means—even though they be entirely new. As a matter of fact, such a method of action often redounds to the good of the patient himself. Pope Pius XII, speaking on September 13, 1952, to the First International Congress on the Histopathology of the Nervous System, said in regard to this point,

---

[54] Kelly, *Medico-Moral Problems*, V, p. 14–15

Without doubt, before the employment of new methods can be morally permitted, one cannot demand that every danger and every risk be excluded. This goes beyond human possibilities; it would paralyze all serious scientific research and would return, very often, to the detriment of the patient. The estimate of the danger ought to be left in these cases to the judgment of the experienced and competent doctor. There exists, nonetheless, and Our explanations have demonstrated it, a series of dangers which morality cannot allow to be caused. It can happen in some dubious cases, all known means having failed, that a new method, still insufficiently tested, will offer, besides the very dangerous elements, good probability of success. If the sick person gives his assent, the application of the procedure in question is licit. But this manner of procedure cannot be established as the norm of conduct for normal cases.[55]

---

[55] "Sans doute, avant d'autoriser en morale l'emploi de nouvelles méthodes, on ne peut exiger que tout danger, tout risque soient exclus. Cela dépasse les possibilités humaines, paralyserait toute recherche scientifique serieuse, et tournerait tres souvent au détriment du patient. L'appréciation du danger doit être laissée dans ces cas au judgement du médecin expérimenté et compétent. Il y a cependant, nos explications l'ont montré, un degré de danger que la morale ne peut permettre. Il peut arriver, dans des cas douteux, quand échouent les moyens déjà connus, qu'une méthode nouvelle, encore insuffisamment éprouvée, offre, à côté d'éléments très dangereu, des chances appréciables de succès. Si le patient donne son accord, l'application du procédé en question est licite. Mais cette manière de faire ne peut être érigée en ligne de conduite pour les cas normaux." Pius XII, Address to the First International Congress on the Histopathology of the Nervous System, September 14, 1952. The original text is taken from *Discorsi e Radiomessaggi di Sua Santità Pio XII* (Vatican City: Typographia Polyglotta Vaticana, 1953), XIV, pp. 329–330.

Here again we note that an essential factor in this problem is the necessity of obtaining the patient's consent. A doctor may use a new method when all known and sure methods have failed, provided that the new method offers some good probability of success and provided that the patient freely consents to the use of the new method. Furthermore, it is necessary to emphasize that the doctor must fully apprise the patient of the risk and dangers involved in the new procedure before he obtains the patient's consent. If the patient refuses to submit to the new cure or the new medical procedure, then neither the doctor's professional ideal nor the common good requires him to employ such a new cure or procedure.

The doctor therefore stands between his patient and his profession. In the last analysis, however, it is his patient that should be his prime concern. The doctor should treat the human being. He should reasonably judge what will bring about the greater good for his patient in accordance with his professional ideal and the patient's wishes, and then the doctor should feel free to follow out his judgment.

SUMMARY POINTS

1. God retains the radical possession of the rights over man's life. Man has full rights to the *use* of his life but to this only. Hence, any form of non-conservation of self, directly intended by an individual on his own authority, is illicit.

2. Likewise, man has the serious positive obligation of caring for his bodily life and health.

3. It is possible that an individual could be invincibly ignorant of this obligation for a time, but certainly not for any extended length of time. However, it is possible that he might realize his obligation to conserve his life but err in the practical application of the obligation to his status here and now.

4. There is no licit application of *epikeia* (reasonable exception) in this matter. Neither is a dispensation possible.

However, an individual could receive the command from God to take his own life by some form of non-conservation of self. In such a case, the individual would then have permission to exercise a faculty ordinarily reserved as a divine prerogative.

5. The obligation to conserve one's life, being an affirmative precept of the natural law, does not require fulfillment under all circumstances. Hence, a moral impossibility would excuse.

6. The means to fulfill this precept of self-conservation are obligatory. Those means binding everyone in common circumstances are ordinary means. Those means involving a moral impossibility are extraordinary means.

7. There is a clear distinction between *natural* means of conserving life and *artificial* means of conserving life. Natural means of conserving life are *per se* intended by nature as the basic means whereby man is to conserve his life, whereas artificial means of conserving life are *per se* intended by nature as a means whereby man can *supplement* the natural means of conserving life. Both the natural means and the artificial means of conserving life are obligatory if they are *ordinary* means of conserving life.

8. There is a clear distinction between the terms "ordinary means of conserving life" and "ordinary medical procedures." What is clearly an ordinary medical procedure is not necessarily an ordinary means of conserving life in the theological sense.

9. The elements used by the moralists in their descriptions of the term, "ordinary means" are: *spes salutis* (hope of benefit), *media communia* (means in common use), *secundum proportionem status* (in keeping with one's status), *media non difficilia* (not too difficult means), and *media facilia* (reasonably simple means).

10. The elements used by the moralists in their descriptions of the term "extraordinary means" are *quaedam impos-*

sibilitas (a certain impossibility), *summus labor* (great effort), *media nimis dura* (excessive hardship), *quidam cruciatus* (excruciating pain), *ingens dolor* (excessive pain), *sumptus extraordinarius* (extraordinary expense), *media pretiosa* (high-priced means), *media exquisita* (the very best means), and *vehemens horror* (intense fear or repugnance).

11. A *relative norm* suffices in determining a means as an ordinary or an extraordinary means of conserving life.

12. There is no *absolute norm* according to which certain means of conserving life are clearly *ordinary* for all men. A relative norm must be applied.

13. It does seem that an *absolute norm* can be established according to which certain means of conserving life are clearly *extraordinary* means of conserving life.

14. It would be allowable to establish a *general norm* in regard to *ordinary* means, by which certain means of conserving life are characterized as ordinary means of conserving life for most men.

15. *Ordinary means of conserving life* may be defined as those means commonly used in given circumstances which this individual in his present physical, psychological, and economic condition can reasonably employ with definite hope of proportionate benefit.

16. *Extraordinary means of conserving life* may be defined as those means not commonly used in given circumstances or those means in common use which this individual in his present physical, psychological, and economic condition cannot reasonably employ, or if he can, will not give him definite hope of proportionate benefit.

17. Ordinary means of conserving life, understood according to the above definition, are always morally obligatory.

18. Extraordinary means of conserving life *per se* are not morally obligatory; however, *per accidens* a particular individual may be bound to employ such means.

19. Even though advances in the field of medical science have reduced greatly the risk involved in surgical interventions, the element of risk must still be considered today in determining surgical procedures as ordinary and extraordinary means, particularly in cases involving patients of advanced age and patients in a weakened physical condition.

20. Concerning operating technique alone: (a) Common surgical interventions, even major ones, performed on patients of young age and relatively strong physical constitution and in surroundings which offer the advantages of modern hospital skill, precautions, and equipment are *generally* ordinary means of conserving life. (b) Major surgical interventions, even common ones, performed on patients of advanced age or of relatively weak constitution, cannot be classed *generally* as ordinary means of conserving life. (c) Major surgical interventions, even common ones, performed on the young or the old in surroundings which do not offer the advantages of modern hospital skill, precautions, and equipment cannot be classed *generally* as ordinary means of conserving life. (d) Radical surgery which involves great risk and danger or which is still insufficiently known is an extraordinary means of conserving life for both the young and the old.

21. The amputation of a leg probably remains an extraordinary means of conserving life, owing to subjective abhorrence. This is certainly true in the case of the amputation of both legs.

22. The basic medicines, intravenous feedings, insulin, the many types of antibiotics, oxygen masks and tents, preventive medicines and vaccines, and blood transfusions are *generally* ordinary means of conserving life.

23. *Per se,* the doctor has the obligation of using the ordinary means of conserving life when he treats a patient *ex caritate* or *ex justitia.* A proportionately grave inconvenience excuses from this obligation.

24. The doctor must employ the extraordinary means of conserving life which the patient, accepted *ex justitia,* is bound to employ or reasonably wishes the doctor to use.

25. Extraordinary means must be used by the doctor in the case of the patient *ex caritate* who needs and wishes such measures, provided the doctor can furnish them without a proportionately grave inconvenience to himself.

26. If the wishes of a patient *ex caritate* in regard to the use of extraordinary means are entirely unknown and a reasonable investigation will not reveal these wishes, the doctor need not employ the extraordinary means of conserving life.

27. If the wishes of a patient *ex justitia* in regard to the use of extraordinary means are entirely unknown and cannot be determined after a reasonable investigation, the doctor, by virtue of his contract with the patient, should make a prudent decision in this regard in the name of the patient which will effect the greater good for the patient.

28. The doctor should feel free in conscience to use or neglect, according to the circumstances of each case, relatively useless artificial life-sustainers.

29. The doctor does not have the obligation of using all means in his power to sustain life, nor does he have the obligation in all circumstances of prolonging life until such prolongation is no longer possible.

30. The doctor must try to effect a cure as long as there is any reasonable hope of doing so.

31. The doctor must try to find a remedy for disease. Hence, he may employ extraordinary means of conserving life, even hitherto insufficiently tested procedures, provided that all known and secure measures have failed, the new procedure gives good probability of success, and he obtains the patient's consent.

Appendices

Pope Pius XII
November 24, 1957

Address to an International Congress of Anesthesiologists on the Prolongation of Life

Dr. Bruno Haid, chief of the anesthesia section at the surgery clinic of the University of Innsbruck, has submitted to Us three questions on medical morals treating the subject known as "resuscitation" [*la réanimation*].

We are pleased, gentlemen, to grant this request, which shows your great awareness of professional duties, and your will to solve in the light of the principles of the Gospel the delicate problems that confront you.

Problems of Anesthesiology

According to Dr. Haid's statement, modern anesthesiology deals not only with problems of analgesia and anesthesia properly so-called, but also with those of "resuscitation." This is the name given in medicine, and especially in anesthesiology, to the technique which makes possible the remedying of certain occurrences which seriously threaten human life, especially asphyxia, which formerly, when modern anesthetizing equipment was not yet available, would stop the heartbeat and bring about death in a few minutes. The task of the anesthesiologist has therefore extended to acute respiratory difficulties, provoked by strangulation or by open wounds of the chest. The anesthesiologist intervenes to prevent asphyxia resulting from the internal obstruction

The English text presented here was originally published in *The Pope Speaks* 4.4 (Spring 1958): 393–398, based on the French text reported in *L'Osservatore Romano*, November 25–26, 1957. The translation is based on one released by the NCWC News Service.

of breathing passages by the contents of the stomach or by drowning, to remedy total or partial respiratory paralysis in cases of serious tetanus, of poliomyelitis, of poisoning by gas, sedatives, or alcoholic intoxication, or even in cases of paralysis of the central respiratory apparatus caused by serious trauma of the brain.

The Practice of "Resuscitation"

In the practice of resuscitation and in the treatment of persons who have suffered head wounds, and sometimes in the case of persons who have undergone brain surgery or of those who have suffered trauma of the brain through anoxia and remain in a state of deep unconsciousness, there arise a number of questions that concern medical morality and involve the principles of the philosophy of nature even more than those of analgesia.

It happens at times—as in the aforementioned cases of accidents and illnesses, the treatment of which offers reasonable hope of success—that the anesthesiologist can improve the general condition of patients who suffer from a serious lesion of the brain and whose situation at first might seem desperate. He restores breathing either through manual intervention or with the help of special instruments, clears the breathing passages, and provides for the artificial feeding of the patient.

Thanks to this treatment, and especially through the administration of oxygen by means of artificial respiration, a failing blood circulation picks up again and the appearance of the patient improves, sometimes very quickly, to such an extent that the anesthesiologist himself, or any other doctor who, trusting his experience, would have given up all hope, maintains a slight hope that spontaneous breathing will be restored. The family usually considers this improvement an astonishing result and is grateful to the doctor.

If the lesion of the brain is so serious that the patient will very probably, and even most certainly, not survive, the anesthesiologist is then led to ask himself the distressing question as to the value and meaning of the resuscitation processes. As an immediate measure he will apply artificial respiration by intubation and by aspiration of the respiratory tract; he is then in a safer position and has more time to decide what further must be done. But he can find himself in a delicate position, if the family considers that the efforts he has taken are improper and opposes them. In most cases this situation arises, not at the beginning of resuscitation attempts, but when the patient's condition, after a slight improvement at first, remains stationary and it becomes clear that only automatic artificial respiration is keeping him alive. The question then arises if one must, or if one can, continue the resuscitation process despite the fact that the soul may already have left the body.

The solution to this problem, already difficult in itself, becomes even more difficult when the family—themselves Catholic perhaps—insist that the doctor in charge, especially the anesthesiologist, remove the artificial respiration apparatus in order to allow the patient, who is already virtually dead, to pass away in peace.

A Fundamental Problem

Out of this situation there arises a question that is fundamental from the point of view of religion and the philosophy of nature. When, according to Christian faith, has death occurred in patients on whom modern methods of resuscitation have been used? Is Extreme Unction valid, at least as long as one can perceive heartbeats, even if the vital functions properly so-called have already disappeared, and if life depends only on the functioning of the artificial respiration apparatus?

Three Questions

The problems that arise in the modern practice of resuscitation can therefore be formulated in three questions:

First, does one have the right, or is one even under the obligation, to use modern artificial-respiration equipment in all cases, even those which, in the doctor's judgment, are completely hopeless?

Second, does one have the right, or is one under obligation, to remove the artificial-respiration apparatus when, after several days, the state of deep unconsciousness does not improve if, when it is removed, blood circulation will stop within a few minutes? What must be done in this case if the family of the patient, who has already received the last sacraments, urges the doctor to remove the apparatus? Is Extreme Unction still valid at this time?

Third, must a patient plunged into unconsciousness through central paralysis, but whose life—that is to say, blood circulation—is maintained through artificial respiration, and in whom there is no improvement after several days, be considered *de facto* or even *de jure* dead? Must one not wait for blood circulation to stop, in spite of the artificial respiration, before considering him dead?

Basic Principles

We shall willingly answer these three questions. But before examining them, We would like to set forth the principles that will allow formulation of the answer.

Natural reason and Christian morals say that man (and whoever is entrusted with the task of taking care of his fellowman) has the right and the duty in case of serious illness to take the necessary treatment for the preservation of life and health. This duty that one has toward himself, toward God, toward the human community, and in most cases toward certain determined persons, derives from well-ordered charity, from submission to the Creator, from social justice and even from strict justice, as well as from devotion toward one's family.

But normally one is held to use only ordinary means—according to circumstances of persons, places, times, and culture—that is to say, means that do not involve any grave burden for oneself or another. A more strict obligation would be too burdensome for most men and would render the attainment of the higher, more important good too difficult. Life, health, all temporal activities are in fact subordinated to spiritual ends. On the other hand, one is not forbidden to take more than the strictly necessary steps to preserve life and health, as long as he does not fail in some more serious duty.

Administration of the Sacraments

Where the administration of sacraments to an unconscious man is concerned, the answer is drawn from the doctrine and practice of the Church which, for its part, follows the Lord's will as its rule of action. Sacraments are meant, by virtue of divine institution, for men of this world who are in the course of their earthly life, and, except for baptism itself, presupposed prior baptism of the recipient. He who is not a man, who is not yet a man, or is no longer a man, cannot receive the sacraments. Furthermore, if someone expresses his refusal, the sacraments cannot be administered to him against his will. God compels no one to accept sacramental grace.

When it is not known whether a person fulfills the necessary conditions for valid reception of the sacraments, an effort must be made to solve the doubt. If this effort fails, the sacrament will be conferred under at least a tacit condition (with the phrase *Si capax est*, "If you are capable," which is the broadest condition). Sacraments are instituted by Christ for men in order to save their souls. Therefore, in cases of extreme necessity, the Church tries extreme solutions in order to give man sacramental grace and assistance.

The Fact of Death

The question of the fact of death and that of verifying the fact itself (*de facto*) or its legal authenticity (*de jure*) have, because of their consequences, even in the field of morals and of religion, an even greater importance. What We have just said about the presupposed essential elements for the valid reception of a sacrament has shown this. But the importance of the question extends also to effects in matters of inheritance, marriage and matrimonial processes, benefices (vacancy of a benefice), and to many other questions of private and social life.

It remains for the doctor, and especially the anesthesiologist, to give a clear and precise definition of "death" and the "moment of death" of a patient who passes away in a state of unconsciousness. Here one can accept the usual concept of complete and final separation of the soul from the body; but in practice one must take into account the lack of precision of the terms "body" and "separation." One can put aside the possibility of a person being buried alive, for removal of the artificial respiration apparatus must necessarily bring about stoppage of blood circulation and therefore death within a few minutes.

In case of insoluble doubt, one can resort to presumptions of law and of fact. In general, it will be necessary to presume that life remains, because there is involved here a fundamental right received from the Creator, and it is necessary to prove with certainty that it has been lost.

We shall now pass to the solution of the particular questions.

A Doctor's Rights and Duties

1. Does the anesthesiologist have the right, or is he bound, in all cases of deep unconsciousness, even in those that are considered to be completely hopeless in the opinion

of the competent doctor, to use modern artificial respiration apparatus, even against the will of the family?

In ordinary cases one will grant that the anesthesiologist has the right to act in this manner, but he is not bound to do so, unless this becomes the only way of fulfilling another certain moral duty.

The rights and duties of the doctor are correlative to those of the patient. The doctor, in fact, has no separate or independent right where the patient is concerned. In general he can take action only if the patient explicitly or implicitly, directly or indirectly, gives him permission. The technique of resuscitation which concerns us here does not contain anything immoral in itself. Therefore the patient, if he were capable of making a personal decision, could lawfully use it and, consequently, give the doctor permission to use it. On the other hand, since these forms of treatment go beyond the ordinary means to which one is bound, it cannot be held that there is an obligation to use them nor, consequently, that one is bound to give the doctor permission to use them.

The rights and duties of the family depend in general upon the presumed will of the unconscious patient if he is of age and sui juris. Where the proper and independent duty of the family is concerned, they are usually bound only to the use of ordinary means.

Consequently, if it appears that the attempt at resuscitation constitutes in reality such a burden for the family that one cannot in all conscience impose it upon them, they can lawfully insist that the doctor should discontinue these attempts, and the doctor can lawfully comply. There is not involved here a case of direct disposal of the life of the patient, nor of euthanasia in any way: this would never be licit. Even when it causes the arrest of circulation, the interruption of attempts at resuscitation is never more than an indirect cause of the cessation of life, and one must apply in this case the principle of double effect and of "*voluntarium in causa.*"

APPENDICES

Extreme Unction

2. We have, therefore, already answered the second question in essence: "Can the doctor remove the artificial respiration apparatus before the blood circulation has come to a complete stop? Can he do this, at least, when the patient has already received Extreme Unction? Is this Extreme Unction valid when it is administered at the moment when circulation ceases, or even after?"

We must give an affirmative answer to the first part of this question, as We have already explained. If Extreme Unction has not yet been administered, one must seek to prolong respiration until this has been done. But as far as concerns the validity of Extreme Unction at the moment when blood circulation stops completely or even after this moment, it is impossible to answer yes or no.

If, as in the opinion of doctors, this complete cessation of circulation means a sure separation of the soul from the body, even if particular organs go on functioning, Extreme Unction would certainly not be valid, for the recipient would certainly not be a man anymore. And this is an indispensable condition for the reception of the sacraments.

If, on the other hand, doctors are of the opinion that the separation of the soul from the body is doubtful, and that this doubt cannot be solved, the validity of Extreme Unction is also doubtful. But, applying her usual rules: "The sacraments are for men" and "In case of extreme measures" the Church allows the sacrament to be administered conditionally in respect to the sacramental sign.

When Is One "Dead"?

3. "When the blood circulation and the life of a patient who is deeply unconscious because of a central paralysis are maintained only through artificial respiration, and no improvement is noted after a few days, at what time does the Catholic Church consider the patient 'dead' or when must

he be declared dead according to natural law (questions *de facto* and *de jure*)?"

(Has death already occurred after grave trauma of the brain, which has provoked deep unconsciousness and central breathing paralysis, the fatal consequences of which have nevertheless been retarded by artificial respiration? Or does it occur, according to the present opinion of doctors, only when there is complete arrest of circulation despite prolonged artificial respiration?)

Where the verification of the fact in particular cases is concerned, the answer cannot be deduced from any religious and moral principle and, under this aspect, does not fall within the competence of the Church. Until an answer can be given, the question must remain open. But considerations of a general nature allow us to believe that human life continues for as long as its vital functions—distinguished from the simple life of organs—manifest themselves spontaneously or even with the help of artificial processes. A great number of these cases are the object of insoluble doubt, and must be dealt with according to the presumptions of law and of fact of which We have spoken.

May these explanations guide you and enlighten you when you must solve delicate questions arising in the practice of your profession. As a token of divine favors which We call upon you and all those who are dear to you, We heartily grant you Our Apostolic Blessing.

⁂

Congregation for the Doctrine of the Faith
May 5, 1980

Declaration on Euthanasia

The rights and values pertaining to the human person occupy an important place among the questions discussed today. In this regard, the Second Vatican Ecumenical Council solemnly reaffirmed the lofty dignity of the human person, and in a special way his or her right to life. The council therefore condemned crimes against life "such as any type of murder, genocide, abortion, euthanasia, or willful suicide" (Pastoral Constitution *Gaudium et Spes*, n. 27).

More recently, the Sacred Congregation for the Doctrine of the Faith has reminded all the faithful of Catholic teaching on procured abortion.[1] The congregation now considers it opportune to set forth the Church's teaching on euthanasia.

It is indeed true that, in this sphere of teaching, the recent popes have explained the principles, and these retain their full force[2]; but the progress of medical science in recent years has brought to the fore new aspects of the question of euthanasia, and these aspects call for further elucidation on the ethical level.

In modern society, in which even the fundamental values of human life are often called into question, cultural change exercises an influence upon the way of looking at suffering and death; moreover, medicine has increased its capacity to cure and to prolong life in particular circumstances, which sometimes give rise to moral problems.

Thus people living in this situation experience no little anxiety about the meaning of advanced old age and death. They also begin to wonder whether they have the right to obtain for themselves or their fellow men an "easy death,"

The English text presented here corresponds to the U.S. Catholic Conference edition of the Vatican text, June 1980.

[1] *Declaration on Procured Abortion*, November 18, 1974: AAS 66 (1974), pp. 730–747.

[2] Pius XII, Address to those attending the Congress of the International Union of Catholic Women's Leagues, September 11, 1947: *AAS* 39 (1947), pp. 2483; Address to the Italian Catho-

which would shorten suffering and which seems to them more in harmony with human dignity.

A number of episcopal conferences have raised questions on this subject with the Sacred Congregation for the Doctrine of the Faith. The congregation, having sought the opinion of experts on the various aspects of euthanasia, now wishes to respond to the bishops' questions with the present declaration, in order to help them to give correct teaching to the faithful entrusted to their care, and to offer them elements for reflection that they can present to the civil authorities with regard to this very serious matter.

The considerations set forth in the present document concern in the first place all those who place their faith and hope in Christ, who, through his life, death, and resurrection, has given a new meaning to existence and especially to the death of the Christian, as St. Paul says: "If we live, we live to the Lord; and if we die, we die to the Lord" (Rom. 14:8; cf. Phil. 1:20).

As for those who profess other religions, many will agree with us that faith in God the Creator, Provider, and Lord of life—if they share this belief—confers a lofty dignity upon every human person and guarantees respect for him or her.

---

lic Union of Midwives, October 29, 1951: *AAS* 43 (1951), pp. 835–854; Speech to the Members of the International Office of Military Medicine Documentation, October 19, 1953: *AAS* 45 (1953), pp. 744–754; Address to Those Taking Part in the Ninth Congress of the Italian Anaesthesiological Society, February 24, 1957: *AAS* 49 (1957), p. 146; cf. also Address on "Reanimation," November 24, 1957: *AAS* 49 (1957), pp. 1027–1033; Paul VI, Address to the Members of the United Nations Special Committee on Apartheid, May 22, 1974: *AAS* 66 (1974), p. 346; John Paul II: Address to the Bishops of the United States of America, October 5, 1979: *AAS* 71 (1979), p. 1225.

It is hoped that this declaration will meet with the approval of many people of good will, who, philosophical or ideological differences notwithstanding, have nevertheless a lively awareness of the rights of the human person. These rights have often, in fact, been proclaimed in recent years through declarations issued by international congresses[3]; and since it is a question here of fundamental rights inherent in every human person, it is obviously wrong to have recourse to arguments from political pluralism or religious freedom in order to deny the universal value of those rights.

I. The Value of Human Life

Human life is the basis of all goods, and is the necessary source and condition of every human activity and of all society. Most people regard life as something sacred and hold that no one may dispose of it at will, but believers see in life something greater, namely, a gift of God's love, which they are called upon to preserve and make fruitful. And it is this latter consideration that gives rise to the following consequences:

1. No one can make an attempt on the life of an innocent person without opposing God's love for that person, without violating a fundamental right, and therefore without committing a crime of the utmost gravity.[4]

2. Everyone has the duty to lead his or her life in accordance with God's plan. That life is entrusted to

---

[3] One thinks especially of recommendation 779 (1976) on the rights of the sick and dying, of the Parliamentary Assembly of the Council of Europe at its 25th Ordinary Session; cf. Sipeca, no. 1, March 1977, 14–15.

[4] We leave aside completely the problems of the death penalty and of war, which involve specific considerations that do not concern the present subject.

the individual as a good that must bear fruit already here on earth, but that finds its full perfection only in eternal life.

3. Intentionally causing one's own death, or suicide, is therefore equally as wrong as murder; such an action on the part of a person is to be considered as a rejection of God's sovereignty and loving plan. Furthermore, suicide is also often a refusal of love for self, the denial of a natural instinct to live, a flight from the duties of justice and charity owed to one's neighbor, to various communities or to the whole of society although, as is generally recognized, at times there are psychological factors present that can diminish responsibility or even completely remove it.

However, one must clearly distinguish suicide from that sacrifice of one's life whereby for a higher cause, such as God's glory, the salvation of souls, or the service of one's brethren, a person offers his or her own life or puts it in danger (cf. Jn 15:14).

II. Euthanasia

In order that the question of euthanasia can be properly dealt with, it is first necessary to define the words used.

Etymologically speaking, in ancient times euthanasia meant an easy death without severe suffering. Today one no longer thinks of this original meaning of the word, but rather of some intervention of medicine whereby the suffering of sickness or of the final agony are reduced, sometimes also with the danger of suppressing life prematurely. Ultimately, the word euthanasia is used in a more particular sense to mean "mercy killing," for the purpose of putting an end to extreme suffering, or having abnormal babies, the mentally ill, or the incurably sick from the prolongation, perhaps for many years, of a miserable life, which could impose too heavy a burden on their families or on society. It is, therefore, necessary to state clearly in what sense the word is used in the present document.

By euthanasia is understood an action or an omission which of itself or by intention causes death, in order that all suffering may in this way be eliminated. Euthanasia's terms of reference, therefore, are to be found in the intention of the will and in the methods used.

It is necessary to state firmly once more that nothing and no one can in any way permit the killing of an innocent human being, whether a fetus or an embryo, an infant or an adult, an old person, or one suffering from an incurable disease, or a person who is dying. Furthermore, no one is permitted to ask for this act of killing, either for himself or herself or for another person entrusted to his or her care, nor can he or she consent to it, either explicitly or implicitly. Nor can any authority legitimately recommend or permit such an action. For it is a question of the violation of the divine law, an offense against the dignity of the human person, a crime against life, and an attack on humanity.

It may happen that, by reason of prolonged and barely tolerable pain, for deeply personal or other reasons, people may be led to believe that they can legitimately ask for death or obtain it for others. Although in these cases the guilt of the individual may be reduced or completely absent, nevertheless the error of judgment into which the conscience falls, perhaps in good faith, does not change the nature of this act of killing, which will always be in itself something to be rejected. The pleas of gravely ill people who sometimes ask for death are not to be understood as implying a true desire for euthanasia; in fact, it is almost always a case of an anguished plea for help and love. What a sick person needs, besides medical care, is love, the human and supernatural warmth with which the sick person can and ought to be surrounded by all those close to him or her, parents and children, doctors and nurses.

III. The Meaning of Suffering for
Christians and the Use of Painkillers

Death does not always come in dramatic circumstances after barely tolerable sufferings. Nor do we have to think only of extreme cases. Numerous testimonies which confirm one another lead one to the conclusion that nature itself has made provision to render more bearable at the moment of death separations that would be terribly painful to a person in full health. Hence it is that a prolonged illness, advanced old age, or a state of loneliness or neglect can bring about psychological conditions that facilitate the acceptance of death.

Nevertheless the fact remains that death, often preceded or accompanied by severe and prolonged suffering, is something which naturally causes people anguish.

Physical suffering is certainly an unavoidable element of the human condition; on the biological level, it constitutes a warning of which no one denies the usefulness; but, since it affects the human psychological makeup, it often exceeds its own biological usefulness and so can become so severe as to cause the desire to remove it at any cost.

According to Christian teaching, however, suffering, especially suffering during the last moments of life, has a special place in God's saving plan; it is in fact a sharing in Christ's passion and a union with the redeeming sacrifice which He offered in obedience to the Father's will. Therefore, one must not be surprised if some Christians prefer to moderate their use of painkillers, in order to accept voluntarily at least a part of their sufferings and thus associate themselves in a conscious way with the sufferings of Christ crucified (cf. Matt. 27:34).

Nevertheless it would be imprudent to impose a heroic way of acting as a general rule. On the contrary, human and Christian prudence suggest for the majority of sick people the use of medicines capable of alleviating or suppressing pain, even though these may cause as a secondary effect semi-consciousness and reduced lucidity. As for those who are not in a state to express themselves, one can reasonably presume that they wish to take these painkillers, and have them administered according to the doctor's advice.

But the intensive use of painkillers is not without difficulties, because the phenomenon of habituation generally makes it necessary to increase their dosage in order to maintain their efficacy. At this point it is fitting to recall a declaration by Pius XII, which retains its full force; in answer to a group of doctors who had put the question: "Is the suppression of pain and consciousness by the use of narcotics ... permitted by religion and morality to the doctor and the patient (even at the approach of death and if one foresees that the use of narcotics will shorten life)?"

The pope said: "If no other means exist, and if, in the given circumstances, this does not prevent the carrying out of other religious and moral duties: Yes."[5] In this case, of course, death is in no way intended or sought, even if the risk of it is reasonably taken; the intention is simply to relieve pain effectively, using for this purpose painkillers available to medicine.

However, painkillers that cause unconsciousness need special consideration. For a person not only has to be able to satisfy his or her moral duties and family obligations; he or she also has to prepare himself or herself with full consciousness for meeting Christ. Thus Pius XII warns: "It is not right to deprive the dying person of consciousness without a serious reason."[6]

---

[5] Pius XII, Address of February 24, 1957: *AAS* 49 (1957), p. 147.

[6] Pius XII, ibid., p. 145; cf. Address of September 9, 1958: *AAS* 50 (1958): 694.

IV. Due Proportion in the
Use of Remedies

Today it is very important to protect, at the moment of death, both the dignity of the human person and the Christian concept of life, against a technological attitude that threatens to become an abuse.

Thus, some people speak of a "right to die," which is an expression that does not mean the right to procure death either by one's own hand or by means of someone else, as one pleases, but rather the right to die peacefully with human and Christian dignity. From this point of view, the use of therapeutic means can sometimes pose problems.

In numerous cases, the complexity of the situation can be such as to cause doubts about the way ethical principles should be applied. In the final analysis, it pertains to the conscience either of the sick person, or of those qualified to speak in the sick person's name, or of the doctors, to decide, in the light of moral obligations and of the various aspects of the case.

Everyone has the duty to care for his or her own health or to seek such care from others. Those whose task it is to care for the sick must do so conscientiously and administer the remedies that seem necessary or useful.

However, is it necessary in all circumstances to have recourse to all possible remedies?

In the past, moralists replied that one is never obliged to use "extraordinary" means. This reply, which as a principle still holds good, is perhaps less clear today, by reason of the imprecision of the term and the rapid progress made in the treatment of sickness. Thus some people prefer to speak of "proportionate" and "disproportionate" means.

In any case, it will be possible to make a correct judgment as to the means by studying the type of treatment to be used, its degree of complexity or risk, its cost and the possibilities of using it, and comparing these elements with the result that can be expected, taking into account the state of the sick person and his or her physical and moral resources.

In order to facilitate the application of these general principles, the following clarifications can be added:

— If there are no other sufficient remedies, it is permitted, with the patient's consent, to have recourse to the means provided by the most advanced medical techniques, even if these means are still at the experimental stage and are not without a certain risk. By accepting them, the patient can even show generosity in the service of humanity.

— It is also permitted, with the patient's consent, to interrupt these means, where the results fall short of expectations. But for such a decision to be made, account will have to be taken of the reasonable wishes of the patient and the patient's family, as also of the advice of the doctors who are specially competent in the matter. The latter may in particular judge that the investment in instruments and personnel is disproportionate to the results foreseen; they may also judge that the techniques applied impose on the patient strain or suffering out of proportion with the benefits which he or she may gain from such techniques.

— It is also permissible to make do with the normal means that medicine can offer. Therefore one cannot impose on anyone the obligation to have recourse to a technique which is already in use but which carries a risk or is burdensome. Such a refusal is not the equivalent of suicide; on the contrary, it should be considered as an acceptance of the human condition, or a wish to avoid the application of a medical procedure disproportionate to the results that can be expected, or a desire not to impose excessive expense on the family or the community.

— When inevitable death is imminent in spite of the means used, it is permitted in conscience to take the decision to refuse forms of treatment that would only secure a precarious and burdensome prolongation of life, so long as the normal care due to the sick person in similar cases is not interrupted. In such circumstances the doctor has no reason to reproach himself with failing to help the person in danger.

Conclusion

The norms contained in the present declaration are inspired by a profound desire to service people in accordance with the plan of the Creator. Life is a gift of God, and on the other hand death is unavoidable; it is necessary, therefore, that we, without in any way hastening the hour of death, should be able to accept it with full responsibility and dignity. It is true that death marks the end of our earthly existence, but at the same time it opens the door to immortal life. Therefore, all must prepare themselves for this event in the light of human values, and Christians even more so in the light of faith.

As for those who work in the medical profession, they ought to neglect no means of making all their skill available to the sick and dying; but they should also remember how much more necessary it is to provide them with the comfort of boundless kindness and heartfelt charity. Such service to people is also service to Christ the Lord, who said: "As you did it to one of the least of these my brethren, you did it to me" (Matt. 25:40).

At the audience granted to the undersigned prefect, his Holiness Pope John Paul II approved this declaration, adopted at the ordinary meeting of the Sacred Congregation for the Doctrine of the Faith, and ordered its publication.

Rome, the Sacred Congregation for the Doctrine of the Faith, May 5, 1980. — Franjo Cardinal Šeper, *Prefect;* Jérôme Hamer, O.P., Titular Archbishop of Lorium, *Secretary*

⅋

Pontifical Council Cor Unum
June 27, 1981

Questions of Ethics regarding the Fatally Ill and the Dying

I. Introduction

1.1. The Working Group

From the 12th to the 14th of November 1976, in keeping with its mandate of coordinating the Activities of the Church in the Health Sector, the Pontifical Council Cor Unum got together a Working Group to study various questions of ethics related to the fatally ill and the dying. The Group was composed of some 15 persons, and was interdisciplinary: there were theologians, doctors, members of Religious Congregations dedicated to the care of the sick, trained nurses, and hospital chaplains.

1.2. The subject discussed by the Working Group

Recent developments in science are influencing medical practice more and more, particularly in the treatment of the fatally ill and the dying. This state of affairs raises prob-

---

The English text presented here corresponds to the text available in 2011 from the Pontifical Academy for Life (http://www .academiavita.org).

lems of a theological and ethical order on which the health professionals are eager to be authoritatively enlightened. Christian members of these professions working in Christian surroundings have long been much concerned about these problems. All the more so are Christians [who are] obliged to work in non-Christian surroundings, and who for this reason desire that their work be inspired by their faith and bear witness to it.

Unfortunately, medical ethics are for many persons a matter of speculation, of more or less accurate information, [and] of erroneous ideas, and all this begets great confusion. COR UNUM is not in a position to undertake a vast programme of doctrinal or scientific research: this is for higher and better qualified authorities. The purpose of our Working Group was simply to analyse basic concepts, point out certain distinctions which must be understood clearly, and formulate practical answers to questions brought up by pastoral directives and by the treatment of the dying.

1.3. The Sacred Congregation for the Doctrine of the Faith

On the 5th of May, 1980, this Congregation published a "Declaration on Euthanasia". In it were authoritatively set forth principles of doctrine and morals on this very serious problem, which has attracted and held the interest of large sectors of the public. As a result, mostly, of special cases that have received wide publicity—cases of what has been called "therapeutic obstinacy"—, people's consciences were aroused and much self-questioning had been going on. This important document first recalls to the reader what the value of human life is, and then proceeds to deal with the subject of euthanasia: it provides Christians with principles for making decisions and taking action where suffering and the use of painkillers are concerned and also where the use of one or another therapeutic treatment is possible.

1.4. Publication of the report on Cor Unum's Working Group

Our 1976 Working Group's reflection is for the most part pastoral: it answers precise and concrete questions put to Cor Unum by hospital chaplains, doctors, and trained nurses. As a result of the publication of the "Declaration on Euthanasia" by the S.C. for the Doctrine of the Faith, our Pontifical Council has been requested to publish the report of its Working Group. Let this be the occasion for us to thank all those who, with a competence deriving only from great experience, contributed to its realization.

2. Fundamental Concepts

2.1. Life

2.1.1. *The Christian meaning of life*

Life is given to mankind by our Creator. It is a gift bestowed in order for man to accomplish a mission. Thus, a person's "right to live" is not what is of foremost importance, since this right is not man's but, rather, belongs to God, who does not give life to human beings as something of which they may dispose as they see fit. Life is directed towards an end towards which it is the responsibility of human beings to direct themselves: towards the perfecting of themselves according to God's plan.

The first corollary of this fundamental concept is that to give up life of one's own choice is to give up striving towards an end which not we but God has established. Mankind has been called upon to make his life useful; he may not destroy it at will. His duty is to care [for] his body, its functions, its organs; to do everything he can to render himself capable of attaining to God. This duty implies giving up things which in themselves may be good. This duty sometimes requires that we sacrifice health and life: our concern for them cannot allow us to deny the claim of superior values. All the same, in the matter of cares to be taken for maintaining good health and preserving life, a correct proportion must be arrived at, regarding both the superior goods perhaps at sake and also the concrete condition in which man lives out his existence on earth.

2.1.2. *We cannot freely dispose of the life of someone else*

If one may not destroy one's life at will, this is also true, a fortiori, of someones else's life. A sick person cannot simply be made the object of decisions which he himself does not make or of which, if he is unable to make them, he would not morally approve. Each human individual, as the person principally responsible for his life, must be at the center of all assistance. Others are present in order to help him, not substitute [for] him. This does not mean, however, that doctors or members of the family may not at times find themselves in the position of having to take decisions for a sick person who for various reasons cannot do so himself, concerning therapeutic measure and treatments to be applied to him. But to the doctors and others in this position, more than to anyone else, it is absolutely forbidden to make an attempt on the life of the patient, even out of compassion and pity.

2.1.3. *The fundamental rights of the human individual*

It is this quintessentially doctrinal subject which the Working Group takes as the basis for its considerations. We are well aware of how immensely difficult it is for those who are not Christians, or who have no belief in a life beyond this life on earth, to give meaning to life and to death. Christians will admit, too, that their position is not specific. But what really is at stake is the defense of the fundamental rights of the human individual. We cannot waver where these are concerned. All the less so, because these rights are so very much in the foreground of political and legislative activity. In order to convince people for whom everything ends at death, of what respect is due their own life and the lives of others, the surest arguments are those which show what consequences are brought about in a society by the lack of rigid measures taken for the protection of human life.

2.2. Death

2.2.1. *The meaning which death has for Christians*

The death of a human being is the end of his corporeal existence. It brings to an end that phase of his divine vocation which is his striving, within the compass of time, towards his total perfection. For a Christian, the moment of death is the moment of his finally being united forever to Christ. Today more than ever, it is pertinent to recall this religious and Christological conception of death. It must go hand in hand with a very real perception of the contingency of our living in our body and of the connection between death and our human condition of being sinners. "For ... whether we live or whether we die, we are the Lord's" (Rom. 14:8). Our attitude towards the dying must be inspired by this conviction, and must not merely be reduced to an effort made by science to put off death as long as possible.

2.2.2. *The right to die a human and dignified death*

Concerning this topic, the members of the Working Group from the Third World emphasized how important it is for a human being to end his days on earth with his personality, as far as possible, whole and entire, both in itself and in its relationships with its milieu, and especially with the family. In countries which are less developed technically and less affected by sophistication, the family gathers round the dying person, and he himself feels a need—almost an essential right—to be thus surrounded. When we observe the conditions required for certain therapies and the total isolation imposed by them upon the sick person, we do not find it out of place to state that the right to die as a human being with dignity demands this social dimension.

2.3. Suffering

2.3.1. *The meaning of "suffering" for a Christian*

Neither suffering nor pain—between which we must be careful to distinguish—is ever to be considered an end in itself. Scientifically speaking, there is still great uncertainty as to what constitutes pain. As for suffering, Christians see in it only Love that can be expressed thereby and the purifying effects which it can have. Pius XII pointed out, in his Allocution of the 24th of February 1957, that suffering which is too intense is likely to keep the mind from maintaining the control it ought to have. We are thus not obliged to think that all pain must be endured at any price or that, stoically, one must not attempt to reduce and calm [it]. The Working Group feels that we can do no better than to refer the reader to the text of Pius XII.

2.3.2. *Effects of suffering and pain*

The capacity for suffering varies from person to person. It is for the doctor, the nurses, and the hospital chaplain (let him not be overlooked!) to determine what spiritual and psychological effects suffering and pain are having on a patient, and to decide whether a certain treatment is to be carried out or not. What the patient says must also be carefully listened to, in order to determine what the real nature of his suffering is: for he, after all, is the best judge of it. Of course a doctor may well think that a patient could have more courage and that he can really put up with more suffering than he believes he can; but the ultimate choice is up to the patient.

2.4. Therapeutic measures

2.4.1. *Ordinary measures and extraordinary measures*

The Working Group considered at some length the distinction between these two kinds of therapies. It is true that the terms are becoming somewhat outmoded in scientific terminology and medical practice, but in theology they are indispensable to the consideration of the validity or invalidity of points of great moral importance. For the theologian applies the term "extraordinary" to measures to which there never exists any obligation to have recourse.

The distinction permits us to draw certain complex realities more closely together. It acts as the "middle term". Life within the compass of time is a basic value but is not an absolute; and we find, consequently, that we must demarcate the limits of the obligation to keep oneself alive. The distinction between "ordinary" and "extraordinary" measures expresses this truth and applies these limits to concrete cases. The use of equivalent terms, particularly the words "care suited to the real needs", perhaps expresses the concept more satisfactorily.

2.4.2. *Criteria for distinguishing*

The criteria whereby we distinguish extraordinary measures from ordinary measures are many. They are to be applied according to each concrete case. Some of them are objective, such as the nature of the measures proposed, how expensive they are, whether it is just to use them, and what options of justice are in the matter of using them. Other criteria are subjective, such as not giving certain patients psychological shocks, anxiety, uneasiness, and so on. It will always be a question, when deciding upon measures to be taken, of establishing to what extent the means to be used and the end being sought are proportionate.

2.4.3. *The criterion of the quality of life: its importance*

Among all the criteria for decision, particular importance must be given to the quality of the life to be saved or kept living by the therapy. The letter of Cardinal Villot to the Congress of the International Federation of Catholic Medical Associations is very clear on this subject: "It must be emphasized that it is the sacred character of life which forbids a physician to kill and makes it a duty for him at the same time to use every resource of his art to fight against death. This does not, however, mean that a physician is under obligation to use all and every one of the life-maintaining techniques offered him by the indefatigable creativity of science. Would it not be a useless torture, in many cases, to impose vegetative reanimation during the last phase of an incurable disease?" (*Documentation Catholique*, 1970, p. 963)

But the criterion of the quality of life is not the only one to be taken into account, since, as we have said above, subjective considerations must enter into a properly cautious judgement as to what therapy to undertake and what therapy not. The fundamental point is that the decision should be made according to rational arguments that have taken well into account the many and various aspects of the situation, including what effect will be had upon the family. The principle to follow is, therefore, that no moral obligation to have recourse to extraordinary measures exists; and that, incidentally, a doctor must follow the wishes of a sick person who refuses the measures.

2.4.4. *Obligatory minimal measures*

On the contrary, there remains the strict obligation to apply under all circumstances those therapeutic measures which are called "minimal": that is, those which are normally and customarily used for the maintenance of life

(alimentation, blood transfusions, injections, etc.). To interrupt these minimal measures would, in practice, be equivalent
to wishing to put an end to the patient's life.

3. Euthanasia

3.1. Inaccuracy of the word "euthanasia"

Historically and etymologically, the word "euthanasia"
means "a peaceful death without suffering and pain". In
present-day usage, the word implies performing an action
or omitting to perform an action with the intent of shortening the life of a patient. This common acceptation of the
word brings into debates about euthanasia a considerable
amount of confusion. It is urgent to clear this up. Documents
on the subject, like those which parliamentary assemblies
have recently been formulating, show what harmful effects
can result from the current lack of precision. Furthermore,
present-day progress in medicine has rendered similarly
ambiguou—and perhaps also superfluous—the distinction
between "active euthanasia" and "passive euthanasia", a distinction that it would be preferable to give up making.

3.2. Actions and decisions which are not
a part of euthanasia

Consequently, the Working Group is of the opinion
that, at least in Catholic milieux, a terminology should be
used which does not include the word "euthanasia" at all:

1. neither to designate the actions involved in terminal
   care which aim at making the last phase of an illness
   less unbearable (rehydration, nursing care, massage,
   palliative medication, keeping the dying person
   company ...);

2. nor to designate the decision to stop certain medical
   therapies which no longer seem to be required by

the condition of the patient. (Traditional language would have expressed this as "decision to give up extraordinary measures".) It is thus not a matter of deciding to let the patient die but, rather, of using technical resources proportionately following a reasonable course suggested by prudence and good judgment;

3. nor to designate an action taken to relieve the suffering of the patient at the risk of perhaps shortening his life. This sort of action is part of a doctor's calling: his vocation is not only that of curing diseases or prolonging life but—much more generally—also that of taking care of a sick person and relieving his suffering.

3.3. The strict meaning of the word

"Euthanasia" must be used only to mean "to put an end to a patient's life by a specific act". Pius XII makes it abundantly clear that, understood in this meaning, euthanasia can never be sanctioned. (Allocution of the 24th of November 1957, *Documentation Catholique*, p. 1609)

Despite the fact that, in practice, the distinctions stated above are sometimes difficult to make, they are nonetheless capable of giving to the word "euthanasia" a meaning free of ambiguities. They can thus be points of reference for the attending physician, who, after consultation with the other doctors and the nurses on the case, with the hospital chaplain, and with the family, will then make his decision.

It will be a decision based upon the principle that neither moral values nor values inherent to the human individual are to be meddled with; that the best judgment concerning what must or must not be done, continued, stopped, or undertaken, will be based upon these values according to each case, and can never be arbitrary.

4. The Use of Painkillers in Terminal Cases

4.1. There are various ways to ease suffering

The use of painkillers affecting the central nervous system involves the risk of secondary effects: they can affect respiratory functions, alter the state of consciousness, cause dependency, and, losing their effect, necessitate larger and larger doses. This is why it is always better not to use them so long as the patient's suffering can be relieved by other means.

These latter are not few in number: remedies such as aspirin, the immobilization of certain parts of the body, various radiation therapies, even surgical operations ... and, above all, combatting the solitude and anguish of the patient simply with the presence of another human being. There are also quite new methods coming into use which enable the patient to acquire a certain mastery of his own body.

4.2. The use of painkillers acting on the central nervous system

In many cases, however, the relief of sometimes truly unbearable suffering does require the use of painkillers acting on the central nervous system (for example, morphine along with other narcotics) at least at the present state of medical knowledge and techniques.

There exists no reason to refuse to make use of such drugs, especially as their side effects can be greatly reduced if they are used judiciously: that is, in appropriate dosages and at accurately determined intervals. For the using of drugs against pain while still keeping the patient as conscious as possible requires a perfect knowledge of these products: the ways to give them, their secondary effects, and their contra-indications. When decisions are being made concerning them, it becomes important for the pharmacologist to be consulted and, even, actually to be with the patient.

4.3. The Necessity of a Human Presence

When speaking of the narcotics, we must warn against the temptation of believing that they are a sufficient remedy for suffering. Human suffering very frequently contains an element of anguish, of fear in the face of the unknown, brought out by severe illness and the nearness of death. Drugs can diminish anguish but, more often than not, are powerless to relieve it completely. It is only a human presence, discreet and attentive, that can procure the relief so much needed, by allowing the sick person to express his thoughts and by giving him human and spiritual comfort.

4.4. Is it permissible to put the sick person into a state of unconsciousness?

We can now approach the question of whether it is right, when death is very near, to use narcotics to put the patient into a state of unconsciousness. In certain cases, the use of them for this purpose is necessary, and Pope Pius XII has recognized the moral rightness of doing so under certain conditions. (Allocution of the 24th of February 1957)

The problem is, however, that there exists a great temptation to have recourse to narcosis as a general practice, doubtless, at times, out of pity, but often more or less deliberately, in order to save the doctors, nurses, family, and others around the patient the emotional wear and tear of being with a person on the verge of death. This clearly indicates that it is not the good of the patient which is being sought; rather, it is the protection of people who are perfectly well but who are members of a society that is afraid of death, that flees death by any means at its disposal.

Yet systematic narcosis deprives the dying patient of the possibility of "living out his death". It deprives him of arriving at a serene acceptance of it; of achieving a state of peace; of sharing, perhaps, a last intense relationship between a person reduced to that last of human poverties and another person who will have been privileged by thus knowing him. And, if the dying person is a Christian, he is being deprived of experiencing his death in communion with Christ.

What is therefore important is to protest vigorously against any systematic plunging into unconsciousness of the fatally ill, and to demand, on the contrary, that medical and nursing personnel learn how to listen to the dying. They must learn how to create relationships among themselves which will sustain them to help families be with their near and dear one during the last phase of life.

4.5. Narcosis and the decision of the patient

The fundamental principle has been laid down, in this entire question, by Pius XII: it must be left to the patient to make decision. "It would be clearly unpermissible to narcotize the dying patient against his express wish (when he is *sui iuris*). If there are serious reasons in favour of deep narcosis, then it must be remembered that the dying person cannot submit to it morally if he has not yet discharged all the duties that are so urgent when life draws to a close". (See below, section 6.1.1.) If the doctor is requested by the patient to give him a deep narcosis, "the doctor will not do so—especially if he is Christian—without first having asked the patient or, better still, having had an intermediary ask him, to fulfill all his duties beforehand". Pius XII goes on to state that, if the dying person refuses to fulfill his duties but still insists upon being narcotized, the doctor may do so: "He may consent to it without making himself guilty of formal collaboration in the sin committed. This sin does not derive from the act of narcotization, but rather from the immoral wish of the patient: for whether he is given narcosis or not, his behaviour will not have changed: he will not have discharged his duties".

5. Cerebral Death

5.1. It is for the science of medicine to define this

In his Allocution of the 24th of November 1957, Pius XII states that "it is for the physician ... to give a clear and precise definition of 'death' and 'the moment of death'". Naturally, we cannot ask of medical science any more than a detailing of criteria whereby it can be established that death has taken place. But what Pius XII means is that it is for medical science and not for the Church to establish these criteria. To the reasons he gives as practical illustrations of his point can today be added requests for organ transplants and the resultant necessity of precisely establishing the donor's moment of death before proceeding to remove the organ to be transplanted.

5.2. The difficulties involved in arriving at this definition

Setting up a medical definition of death is complicated by the fact that, at the present state of our knowledge, death apparently does not take place all at once. It is not an instantaneous cessation of all the functions of the body, but rather a series of cessations of our various life processes, one after the other. It seems that what stops first is the mechanism that regulates the functioning together of all the organs of the body. This mechanism is situated in the brain. After it stops, necrosis then begins to spread to the various systems: the nervous system, the cardiovascular, respiratory, digestive, urogenital, and locomotor systems. And last of all, necrosis reaches the cellular and subcellular components. Yet even today, one cannot be too cautious in this matter, for many uncertainties still exist concerning the "medical definition of death".

There is, however, a growing consensus of opinion that considers a human being dead in whom a total and irreversible absence of life activity in the brain has been established. This is known as "cerebral death". Various authoritative groups have drawn up lists of criteria concerning it. These criteria may not be completely identical, but there is sufficient correspondence among them to make up a list of symptoms of death whose accuracy can be taken as very highly probable. Conventional agreements and administrative procedure are already in effect or are being arrived at, which, if all the required criteria can be demonstared, permit or will permit the release of death certificates and, thereafter, the removal of the organs to be used in transplant operations.

5.3. The Church has been asked for a declaration

On the other hand, families are showing increased reticence in the matter of giving permission for the removal of organs for transplant. The Working Group was informed that this is why certain highly authoritative medical groups have requested the Church to make an official declaration on the validity or non-validity of taking cerebral death, duly established, as the "moment of death" of the human being.

The Working Group feels that it is for a higher authority than itself to make such a declaration officially, but has agreed to call attention, by means of this report, to the need for making it. However, the theologians in the Group point out that, even though the proper ecclesiastical authority complied with the request, the Church would not be able to answer the question merely by making [on?] its own any scientific assertion or, still less, by issuing a list of criteria whereby cerebral death is to be determined. The very most the Church could do would be to reiterate the conditions that would make it legitimate to accept the better judgement of those to whose specific competence has been entrusted the determination of the moment of death.

5.4. Measures to be taken in cases of apparent death

As Pius XII states, it is the physician's duty, in cases of apparent death, to do everything he can do, by every ordinary means, to restore life activity. Nonetheless, a moment always comes when death can be considered as having taken place, and when reanimation measures can be stopped without committing either a professional or a moral eror. (Pius XII, Allocution of the 24th of November 1957).

6. Communicating with Dying People

6.1. The right to know the truth

The communication with dying patients brings up the moral question of their right to know the truth. The clergy, pastorally, and doctors and nurses, professionally, must consider what sort of behaviour a dying person has a right to expect from those around him. The dying and, more generally, anyone with an incurable disease have a right to be told the truth. Death is too essential an event for the envisioning of it to be avoided. In the case of a believer, its approach requires preparation and specific actions made in full consciousness. In the case of any human being, dying brings the responsibility of fulfilling certain duties towards one's family, of putting order to business affairs, bringing accounts up to date, settling debts, etc. In any case, preparation for dying should begin long before the approach of death and while a person is still in good health.

6.1.2. *The responsibility of those surrounding a dying person*

Whoever is nearest the patient must inform him of the possibility of his dying. The family, the chaplain, and the group providing medical care must assume their share in this duty. Each case is different, depending on the sensitivies and capabilities of all concerned, and on the condition of the patient and his ability to relate to others. How he will react to the truth—by rebellion, depression, resignation, and so on—is what those surrounding him must try to foresee, in order to be able to behave with tact and calm. A ray of hope may licitly be held out to the patient; death may even be presented as not 100% certain—but only provided that doing this does not totally conceal the possibility of dying, the serious probability.

6.1.3. *The mission of the hospital chaplain*

Here is where the continuous assistance of the chaplain during the illness has its utmost importance. His mission confers upon him a privileged role in preparing a patient little by little for death. Of course the duty to believe, right to the very end, in the efficacy *ex opere operato* of the sacraments (Confession, Viaticum, and Extreme Unction) and when necessary of giving them conditionally according to canon law, remains untouched. And yet we must point out that the unexpected appearance of the priest at the last moment makes the performance of his ministry very difficult and, at times, impossible. The hospital chaplain will try, therefore, to create, through continual contacts, a relationship of confidence with the patients, especially in milieux where there are lax or indifferent Catholics. He must be careful not to talk of the nearness of death too soon, while at the same time not concealing the truth. The Working Group does not consider it superfluous, furthermore, to insist that, at least in Catholic hospitals and by Catholic doctors and nurses, the chaplain be granted his rightful position, both in consultations about the patient and as one of the persons having access to him at all times.

6.2. Society's attitude towards death

6.2.1. *In the Western World*

Western society today is going through what can only be called "flight in the face of death". Medical and hospital personnel are experiencing this phenomenon and families too. The representatives of the Committee for the Family who took part in our Working Group reported to us some very discomforting examples of the change in attitude towards death within the same families over the course of only 30 years. One case was that of a family which, around 1930, fully took on the death of the mother—even the youngest members; and which, in the 1960s, fled from death, did not even speak of it to children, totally abandoned a dying wife.

We find that, while the medical personnel are trying to put off as long as possible the moment of physiological death under the pretense of calming pain, they are really causing by these measures the greatest anguish and moral suffering in the patient, who, in most cases, is more aware of the seriousness of his condition than those around him affect to think that he is. The dying person feels sadness, guilt, anxiety, fear, and depression, and all of that along with physical pain. Worst of all for him is the isolation, the loneliness, which seriously influence him psychosomatically. The present-day tendency of cutting a dying person off, first from society, then from family, and finally from the other patients in the hospital, deprives him, in his distress, of any and every possibility of communicating with someone else. And there are so many ways to relieve his loneliness, without even taxing him physically: the expression of a human face, a hand to hold! Often merely a silent presence is all he needs, but he needs it with every fibre of his being.

Thus, the practice of Western hospitals in these cases must be revised completely. Even the hospital personnel, for reasons not totally without cause, now tend to protect themselves against what seems a nerve-racking contact: they avoid being with dying patients, whose distress requires the very comfort their presence might give. Once again, it should be a matter for group work—teamwork—to keep the dying from being deprived of this moral support. And doctors, nurses, and chaplains alike must share in this teamwork.

6.2.2. *In other parts of the world*

In other societies, quite to the contrary, we find respect of the patient's right to be assisted by his near and dear, and of the family's right to be with their dying loved ones. Often the family even prefers to remove the dying person from the hospital so that he may be sure to have their presence and, if they are believers, so as to communicate with him through prayer. It is true that sometimes, in the real interest of the patient, doctors must know how to curtail the demands of the family and their insistence upon having the right of decision in the matter of what treatment is to be followed—unless, that is, the patient is a child and thus under parental responsibility. And yet this curtailment should in no way risk fostering the all too real Western tendency of ignoring the family, their presence, and, particularly, their just demands to know the truth.

7. The Responsibilities of Doctors and Nurses

7.1. Necessary knowledge of the medical deontology

It is becoming clearer and clearer that the scientific aspects and the ethical aspects of the medical profession cannot easily be considered separately. If progress in knowledge and techniques is providing a doctor with new instruments and new therapies, the immediate result is that he is often being confronted by ever more complex moral questions.

We have spoken earlier of the fact that it is for the physician, in the last analysis, to make his decision by referring to objective moral criteria. This means, however, that he must have been taught what these criteria are and must have been trained to apply them to specific individual cases. The teaching of moral theory and of codes of medical ethics is rightly, therefore, an essential part of the training of doctors and nurses.

Professors and students must in no way consider such courses as supplementary or "extra" only for those who wish to take them out of curiosity. In countries where there exists a tradition of common law, future physicians are at least encouraged to look into the requirements of moral theory and practice by the very fact that their breaking an ethical and legal precedent would subject them to penal sanctions. But no future physician anywhere should avoid considering the essential interest of patients whom moral law defends and for whom codes of medical ethics have been evolved.

As to the best way to impart these teachings, it can be carried out, on the one hand, in special courses and, on the other, the moral aspects of scientific questions will be treated along with the scientific teaching itself, and thereby illustrated and insisted upon.

7.2. The choice of one therapy or another

As a general rule, and despite what the press leads people to believe, a doctor does not ask himself whether to allow or not allow a patient to die. He decides upon a certain medical treatment: what are its indications, what are its contraindications? These all require him to consider various factors. He does so in the light of moral principles as well as of scientific knowledge. This is how it becomes of great value to a doctor to consider them while he reflects, What must or must not be undertaken? When should extraordinary measures be recurred to and when not? And if so, for what reasons and for how long? Too often, a doctor may come to question himself as to the advisability of continuing a certain treatment, and the question he may put to himself is "Was it wise to have begun the treatment in the first place?" For if there exist moral reasons for prolonging life, there also exist moral reasons for not opposing death with what is known as "therapeutic obstinacy".

7.3. Massive therapy and choosing the persons to receive it

Among the ethical questions brought up by "massive therapies" requiring very highly evolved and expensive equipment and techniques is to be considered the selection of patients to whom to apply a therapy that cannot be applied to everyone with the same malady. Is it legitimate to use the resources of refined medical techniques for the benefit of only one patient, while others are still not receiving the most elementary treatment? One has a right to ask. If certain persons believe that such a question is "going against progress", Christians, at least, should bear it in mind in their valuation.

7.4. Trained nurses, male and female

7.4.1. *The importance of their responsibilities*

Despite the fact that many doctors tend to look upon them as purely auxiliary, nurses have a fundamental role of mediation between doctors and patients. Although nurses are, it is true, by no means free of the danger of avoiding the patient during the final stages of his illness, they are nevertheless responsible for actions that can often be of crucial importance. They must decide, for example, whether or not to call the doctor when they find that the patient has suddenly become worse, or must decide whether or not to give the patient a calming substance the doctor has left it up to their judgement to use at the appropriate moment, etc. Fortunately, in many hospitals today, a true feeling of teamwork between doctors and nurses is beginning to prevail. Their close collaboration is essential to the relief and proper care of each patient.

7.4.2. *Co-operation and conscience*

At times, especially when she or he works in non-Christian hospitals or for non-Christian doctors, the nurse is brought up against a moral dilemma posed by an order given by the doctor, the execution of which would gravely endanger, if not actually put an end to, the patient's life.

First and foremost, the nurse must adhere to the absolute prohibition against performing an act whose only purpose is to kill. Neither the doctor's order, nor the request of the family, nor even the plea of the patient can free the nurse from responsibility for such an act. Where actions are concerned which in themselves are not towards killing (even though the nurse knows that an impermissible result is being aimed at), the case is different if the nurse performs these actions by order of the doctor. Examples of this are doing something which will shorten the life of the patient, suspending a treatment which is not "extraordinary", depriving of consciousness a patient who has not been able to fulfill his obligations. The nurse may not take the initiative for such actions. The only possible way to look at a nurse's performing them is as their being a "material co-operation" excusable only by necessity when examined in the light (1) of the gravity of the action; (2) of the nurse's participation in the whole process and the obtaining of the immoral goal; and (3) of reasons which might have led the nurse to obey the order: fear of something personal being done to her or to him if the order is not carried out; an important personal good [to] be protected by not exposing oneself to the risk of being dismissed. Insofar as her or his status permits, the nurse who finds her or himself involved in practices of which one's conscience cannot approve will make every effort possible to bear witness to her or his personal convictions.

Catholic chaplains and physicians are in duty bound to help nurses face up to such difficult situations, in every way they can.

7.4.3. *Ethical training in nursing schools*

All that we have reported in section 7.1 concerning the necessity of ethical training for doctors, pharmacologists, *et alii,* holds true in the case of nursing schools as well. Catholic nursing schools have the right and the duty to defend, through their teaching, the ethical principles of the Church's Magisterium, particulary in courses which treat of the exercise of the nurse's profession: the value of each human individual, respect for life, morality and marriage, and so on. It is the duty of Catholic nursing schools to make this ethical orientation clear to all students applying for entrance. The schools further have the right to demand of all students their acceptance of these principles and their attendance at courses specializing in the teaching of professional ethics. The students must arrive at the conviction that here is an essential element, a condition *sine qua non,* of the proper training of a responsible nurse. Nor should this teaching be limited to a casuistical presentation of the subject. Rather, the professors will in every way seek to inculcate a profound familiarity with such fundamental notions as life, death, the personal vocation which a nurse has, and so on.

7.4.4. *Training for the nursing of the incurably ill*

The familiarization of hospital personnel with the demands made by death and by the care of the dying does not take place only at the intellectual level. The actual face-to-face ecounter with suffering, with a patient's anxiety, with death, can be a source of great anguish. Here is one of the main reasons why many professional people today are beginning to avoid having anything personal to do with the incurably ill, and are abandoning them to their loneliness. Thus must be added to the teaching of the theory and study of professional ethics, an education in how to relate to people, and especially to the incurably ill. If this is not taught, then any teaching of ethics is in danger, in the long run, of not being applied to the real situations encountered professionally.

8. The Responsibilities of Family and Society

8.1. Education for suffering and death

The ties between life and death have become so very much loosened, at least in our Western society, that death has little by little lost its significance.

The family and the society by which it is surrounded have each their own part in this situation, which can only be considered highly destructive. It is urgent that education about suffering and death be undertaken. This would perhaps be the solution to the numerous problems existing today concerning death and the dying.

8.2. Questions we must ask ourselves

The family must begin to question itself on this subject,

1. in order to see whether suffering, death, failure, etc., are present or absent in its child-education habits, beginning with the earliest ages of life;

2. in order to determine what place it accords to sick persons, the handicapped, people who have failed in life, old people, and the dying.

If it is found that this education and this sharing are not a part of the family ways, if there is no family attitude and habit which are signs of love and of faith in the value of each and every human being, then how can we hope to create the communication so greatly desired between the dying person and his family during the last moments of earthly life?

8.3. Society and the family. Legislation

Society, too, must also ask itself what it is bringing of any value to the family where this educative mission is concerned, whether it be to the family's habitat, to the various kinds of work its members perform, to its health, or to its problems with the sick and the aged.

Above all, we have every cause to be apprehensive lest the family's solidarity with its members who are suffering—and solidarity in every sort of suffering—be gravely threatened by certain kinds of present-day legislation: for example, laws "regulating" divorce, contraception, and abortion and tomorrow, perhaps, euthanasia.

❦

Pope John Paul II
October 21, 1985

Address to the Pontifical Academy of Sciences

Ladies and Gentlemen,

1. I extend a most cordial welcome to all of you. And I rejoice with the Pontifical Academy of Sciences and its illustrious President, Professor Carlos Chagas, for having succeeded in bringing together two groups of such distinguished scientists to reflect on the subject: "The Artificial Prolongation of Life and the Determination of the Exact Moment of Death", and "The Interaction of Parasitic Diseases and Nutrition".

In the specialised areas encompassed by these subjects, the men and women of science and medicine give yet another proof of their desire to work for the good of humanity. The Church is joined with you in this task, for she too seeks to be *the servant of humanity*. As I said in my first Encyclical, *Redemptor Hominis*: "The Church cannot abandon man, for his 'destiny', that is to say, his election, calling, birth and death, salvation or perdition, is so closely and unbreakably linked with Christ".[1]

The English text presented here is from *Papal Addresses to the Pontifical Academy of Sciences 1917–2002 and to the Pontifical Academy of Social Sciences 1994–2002* (Vatican City: PAS, 2003), 271–274.

[1] John Paul II, *Redemptor Hominis*, n. 14.

2. Your presence reminds me of the Gospel parable of the Good Samaritan, the one who cared for an unnamed person who had been stripped of everything by robbers and left wounded at the side of the road. *The figure of that Good Samaritan I see reflected in each one of you*, who by means of science and medicine offer your care to nameless sufferers, both among peoples in full development and among the hosts of those individuals afflicted by diseases caused by malnutrition.

For the Christian, life and death, health and sickness, are given fresh meaning by the words of Saint Paul: "None of us lives for himself, and none of us dies for himself. If we live, we live for the Lord, and if we die, we die for the Lord; so then, whether we live or whether we die, we are the Lord's".[2]

These words offer great meaning and hope to us who believe in Christ; non-Christians, too, whom the Church esteems and with whom she wishes to collaborate, understand that within the mystery of life and death there are values which transcend all earthly treasures.

3. When we approach the subject which you have dealt with in your first Group, "The Artificial Prolongation of Life and the Determination of the Exact Moment of Death", we do so with two fundamental convictions, namely: Life is a treasure; Death is a natural event.

Since *life is indeed a treasure*, it is appropriate that scientists promote research which can enhance and prolong human life and that physicians be well informed of the most advanced scientific means available to them in the field of medicine.

Scientists and physicians are called to place their skill and energy at the service of life. They can never, for any reason or in any case, suppress it. For all who have a keen sense of the supreme value of the human person, believers

---

[2] Rm. 14: 7–8.

and non-believers alike, euthanasia is a crime in which one must in no way cooperate or even consent to. *Scientists and physicians must not regard themselves at the lords of life, but as its skilled and generous servants.* Only God who created the human person with an immortal soul and saved the human body with the gift of the Resurrection is the Lord of life.

4. It is the task of doctors and medical workers to give the sick the treatment which will help to cure them and which will aid them to bear their sufferings with dignity. Even when the sick are incurable they are never untreatable: whatever their condition, appropriate care should be provided for them.

Among the useful and licit forms of treatment is *the use of pain-killers.* Although some people may be able to accept suffering without alleviation, for the majority pain diminishes their moral strength. Nevertheless, when considering the use of these, it is necessary to observe the teaching contained in the Declaration issued on 4 June 1980 by the Congregation for the Doctrine of the Faith: "Painkillers that cause unconsciousness need special consideration. For a person not only has to be able to satisfy his or her moral duties and family obligations; he or she also has to prepare himself or herself with full consciousness for meeting Christ".

5. The physician is not the lord of life, but neither is he the conqueror of death. *Death is an inevitable fact of human life, and the use of means for avoiding it must take into account the human condition.* With regard to the use of ordinary and extraordinary means the Church expressed herself in the following terms in the Declaration which I have just mentioned: "If there are no other sufficient remedies, it is permitted, with the patient's consent, to have recourse to the means provided by the most advanced medical techniques, even if these means are still at the experimental stage and are not without a certain risk. ... It is also permitted, with the patient's consent, to interrupt these means, where the results fall short of expectations. But for such a decision to be made,

account will have to be taken of the reasonable wishes of the patient and the patient's family, as also of the advice of the doctors who are specially competent in the matter ... It is also permissible to make do with the normal means that medicine can offer. Therefore one cannot impose on anyone the obligation to have recourse to a technique which is already in use but which carries a risk or is burdensome ... When inevitable death is imminent in spite of the means used, it is permitted in conscience to take the decision to refuse forms of treatment that would only secure a precarious and burdensome prolongation of life, so long as the normal care due to the sick person in similar cases is not interrupted".

6. We are grateful to you, Ladies and Gentlemen, for having studied in detail the *scientific problems connected with attempting to define the moment of death*. A knowledge of these problems is essential for deciding with a sincere moral conscience the choice of ordinary or extraordinary forms of treatment, and for dealing with the important moral and legal aspects of transplants. It also helps us in the further consideration of whether the home or the hospital is the more suitable place for treatment of the sick and especially of the incurable.

The right to receive good treatment and the right to be able to die with dignity demand human and material resources, at home and in hospital, which ensure the comfort and dignity of the sick. Those who are sick and above all the dying must not lack the affection of their families, the care of doctors and nurses and the support of their friends.

Over and above all human comforts, no one can fail to see the enormous help given to the dying and their families by *faith in God and by hope in eternal life*. I would therefore ask hospitals, doctors and above all relatives, especially in the present climate of secularisation, to make it easy for the sick to come to God, since in their illness they experience new questions and anxieties which only in God can find an answer.

7. In many areas of the world the matter which you have begun to study in your second working group has immense importance, namely *the question of malnutrition*. Here the problem is not merely that of a scarcity of food but also the quality of food, whether it is suitable or not for the healthy development of the whole person. Malnutrition gives rise to diseases which hinder the development of the body and likewise impede the growth and maturity of intellect and will.

The research which has been completed so far and which you are now examining in greater detail in this colloquium aims at identifying and treating the diseases associated with malnutrition. At the same time, it points to the need to adapt and improve methods of cultivation, methods which are capable of producing food with all the elements that can ensure proper human subsistence and the full physical and mental development of the person.

It is my fervent hope and prayer that your deliberations will encourage the governments and peoples of the economically more advanced countries to help the populations more severely affected by malnutrition.

8. Ladies and Gentlemen, the Catholic Church, which in the coming World Synod of Bishops will celebrate the twentieth anniversary of the Second Vatican Council, reconfirms the words which the Council Fathers addressed to the men and women of thought and science: "Our paths could not fail to cross. Your road is ours. Your paths are never foreign to ours. We are the friends of your vocation as searchers, companions in your labours, admirers of your successes, and, if necessary, consolers in your discouragement and your failures.

It is with these sentiments that I invoke the blessings of God, the Lord of life, upon the Pontifical Academy of Sciences, upon all the members of the two present working groups and upon your families.

๛

Pontifical Academy of Sciences
December 5, 1985

Report of a Study Group on the Artificial Prolongation of Life

On the invitation of the Pontifical Academy of Sciences, a study group met October 19–21, 1985, to study "the artificial prolongation of life and the exact determination of the moment of death."

After having noted the recent progress of the techniques of resuscitation and the immediate and long-term effects of brain damage, the study group discussed the objective criteria of death and of the rules of conduct in the face of a persistent state of apparent death. On the one hand, experiments carried out reveal that brain resistance to the absence of cerebral circulation can permit recoveries otherwise deemed impossible.

On the other hand, it has been found that when the entire brain has suffered irreversible damage (cerebral death), all possibility of sensitive and cognitive life is definitively ruled out, while a brief vegetative survival can be maintained by artificial prolongation of respiration and circulation.

1. Definition of Death

A person is dead when he has irreversibly lost all capacity to integrate and coordinate the physical and mental functions of the body.

Death occurs when:

a. The spontaneous cardiac and respiratory functions have definitively ceased; or

---

The English text presented here is from *Origins* 15.25 (December 5, 1985).

b. If an irreversible cessation of every brain function is verified.

From the debate it emerged that cerebral death is the true criterion of death, since the definitive arrest of the cardio-respiratory functions leads very quickly to cerebral death.

The group then analyzed the different clinical and instrumental methods that enable one to ascertain the irreversible arrest of the cerebral functions. To be certain—by means of the electroencephalogram—that the brain has become flat, that is to say, that it no longer displays electric activity, it is necessary that the examination be carried out at least twice at a distance of six hours.

2. Medical Guidelines

By the term treatment the group understands all those medical interventions available and appropriate in a specific case, whatever the complexity of the techniques involved.

If the patient is in a permanent, irreversible coma, as far as can be foreseen, treatment is not required, but all care should be lavished on him, including feeding.

If it is clinically established that there is a possibility of recovery, treatment is required.

If treatment is of no benefit to the patient, it may be interrupted while continuing with the care of the patient.

By the term care the group understands ordinary help due to sick patients, such as compassion and spiritual and affective support due to every human being in danger.

3. Artificial Prolongation of Vegetative Functions

In the case of cerebral death, artificial respiration can prolong the cardiac function for a limited time. This induced survival of the organs is indicated in the case of a foreseen removal of organs for a transplant.

This eventuality is possible only in the case of total and irreversible brain damage occurring in a young person, essentially as a result of a very severe injury.

Taking into consideration the important advances made in surgical techniques and in the means to increase tolerance to transplants, the group holds that transplants deserve the support of the medical profession, of the law and of people in general.

The donation of organs should, in all circumstances, respect the last will of the donor or the consent of the family, if present.

Bibliography

Abelard, Peter. *Theologica et philosophica*. Vol. 178 of *Patrologiae cursus completus*, series latina. Paris: Migne, 1844–1864.

Aertnys, J., and C. Damen. *Theologiae moralis*. 16th ed. Turin: Marietti, 1950.

Alphonsus. *Homo apostolicus*. Turin: Marietti, 1848.

———. *Theologica moralis*. Rome: Typographica Vaticana,1948.

Antonius. *Theologica moralis*. Verona, 1749.

Aquinas, Thomas. *Summa theologiae*. Turin: Marietti, 1950.

———. *Super epistolas S. Pauli*. Turin: Marietti, 1953.

Arregui, A. *Summarium theologiae moralis*, 18th ed. Bilbao: Mensajero, 1948.

Augustine. *City of God*. Translated by Marcus Dods. New York: Random House, 1950.

———. *De civitate Dei*. Vol. 41 of *Patrologiae cursus completus, series latina*. Paris: Migne, 1844–1864.

Ballerini, A. *Opus theologicum morale in Busenbaum medullam*. Edited by D. Palmieri. Prati, 1899.

Bañez, D. *Decisiones de iure et iustitia*. Vol. 4 of *Scholastica commentaria in partem angelici doctoris S. Thomae*. Douai, 1614–1615.

Bender, L. "Organorum humanorum transplantatio." *Angelicum* 31 (April–June 1954): 148–149.

Bertke, S. *The Possibility of Invincible Ignorance of the Natural Law*. Washington, D.C.: Catholic University Press, 1941.

Billuart, C. *Summa S. Thomae*. Paris, 1852.

Bonacina, M. *Moralis theologica*. Lyon, 1645.

Bonnar, A. *The Catholic Doctor*. London: Burns Oates and Washbourne, 1952.

Bucceroni, J. *Institutiones theologiae moralis*, 6th ed. Rome, 1914–1915.

Busenbaum, H. *Medulla theologiae moralis*. Rome, 1757.

Capellmann, C. *Medicina pastoralis*, 13th ed. Aachen, 1901.

Catechismus ex decreto SS Concilii Tridentini. Padua, 1758.

Cathrein, V. *Philosophia moralis*. 20th ed. Freiburg: Herder, 1955.

Clark-Kennedy, A. E. "Medicine in Relation to Society," *British Medical Journal* 1.4914 (March 12, 1955): 619–623.

Code of Canon Law, Latin–English edition. Washington, D.C.:*Code of Ethical and Religious Directives for Catholic Hospitals*. St. Louis: Catholic Hospital Association of the United States and Canada, 1949.

Connell, F. *Morals in Politics and Professions*. Westminster, MD: Newman Press, 1951.

Connery, J. "Notes on Moral Theology." *Theological Studies* 16 (1955): 571.

Costa-Rossetti, J. *Philosophia moralis*. Innsbruck: Rauch, 1886.

Cronin, M. *The Science of Ethics*. Dublin: Gill & Son, 1917.

Cunningham, B. *The Morality of Organic Transplantation*. Washington, D.C.: Catholic University Press, 1944.

Cunningham, R. *The Story of Blue Shield*. New York: Public Affairs Committee, 1954.

Davis, H. *Moral and Pastoral Theology*, 3rd ed. London: Sheed and Ward, 1938.

De Lugo, J. *De iustitia a iure* (Lyon, 1642), disp. X, sec. I, n. 9.

————. *De iustitia a iure*. Vol. 6 of *Disputationes scholasticae et morales*. Paris, 1868–1869.

Diana, A. *Coordinatus*. Edited by Martin de Alcolea. Lyon, 1667.

Dictionnaire de Théologie Catholique . Paris: Letouzey et Ané, 1941.

Donovan, J. "Question Box," *Homiletic and Pastoral Review* 49 (August 1949): 904.

Elbel, B. *Theologia moralis per modum conferentiarum*. Edited by I. Bierbaum. Paderborn, 1891–1892.

Escobar, A. de. *Universae theologiae moralis, receptiores absque lite sententiae nec non controversae disquisitiones*. Lyon, 1663.

Fanfani, L. *Manuale theorico-practicum theologiae moralis*. Rome: Liberaria Ferrari, 1950.

Ferreres, J. *Compendium theologia moralis*, 16th ed. Barcelona: Subirana, 1940.

Ford, J. "The Refusal of Blood Transfusions by Jehovah's Witnesses." *Linacre Quarterly* 22 (February 1955): 3–10.

Gabrielis a S. Vincentio. *De justitia et jure.* Rome, 1663.

Gannon, P. "La Grève de la Faim," *La Documentation Catholique* 30 (1920): 333–336.

Gannon, T. *Psychology: The Unity of Human Behavior.* Boston: Ginn and Co., 1954.

Genicot, E., and I. Salsmans. *Institutiones theologiae moralis*, 17th ed. Brussels: L'Edition Universelle, 1951.

Goodwine, J. "The Physician's Duty to Preserve Life by Extraordinary Means." *Proceedings of the Catholic Theological Society of America* 7 (1952): 125–138.

Gury, J. *Compendium theologiae moralis*, 17th ed. Rome, 1866.

———. *Compendium theologiae moralis.* Edited by A. Ballerini and D. Palmieri. Rome, 1907.

Gustafson, G. *The Theory of Natural Appentency in the Philosophy of St. Thomas.* Washington, D.C.: Catholic University Press, 1944.

Guthrie, D. *A History of Medicine* . London: Nelson & Sons, 1947.

Healy, E. *Moral Guidance.* Chicago: Loyola Univerity Press, 1942.

Holzmann, A. *Theologia moralis.* Benevento, 1743.

Hürth, F. *De statibus.* Rome: Pontificia Universitas Gregoriana, 1946.

Hürth. F., and P. Abellán. *De praeceptis*. Rome: Pontificia Universitas Gregoriana, 1948.

———. *De principiis*. Rome: Pontificia Universitas Gregoriana, 1948.

Iturrioz, Iesus, and others. *Philosophiae scholasticae summa*. Madrid: Biblioteca de Autores Cristianos, 1952.

Jerome. *Commentaria in Jonam*. Vol. 25 of *Patrologiae cursus completus, series latina*. Paris: Migne, 1844–1864.

Jone, H., and U. Adelman. *Moral Theology*. Westminister, MD: Newman Press, 1948.

Jorio, T. *Theologia moralis*, 4th ed. Naples: D'Auria, 1954.

Kelly, G. "The Duty to Preserve Life." *Theological Studies* 12 (December 1951): 550–556.

———. "The Duty of Using Artificial Means of Preserving Life." *Theological Studies* 11 (June 1950): 203–220

———. *Medico-Moral Problems*. St. Louis: Catholic Hospital Association of the U.S. and Canada, 1954.

Lacroix, C. *Theologia moralis*. Ravenna, 1761.

Lactantius, *Divinarum institutionum*. Vol. 6 of *Patrologiae cursus completus, series latina*. Paris: Migne, 1844–1864.

Lanza, A., and P. Palazzini. *Theologia moralis*. Turin: Marietti, 1955.

Laymann, P. *Theologica moralis*. Munich, 1626.

Leclercq, J. *Les droits et devoirs individuels*. Vol. 4 of *Leçons de droit naturel*. Namur: Wesmael-Charlier, 1937.

Lehmkuhl, A. *Theologia moralis*. 10th ed. Freiburg: Herder, 1902.

Leo XIII, *Pastoralis offici*. September 12, 1891. In H. Denzinger, *Enchiridion symbolorum definitionum et declarationum de rebus fidei et morum*. Edited by J. Umberg. Freiburg: Herder, 1942.

Lessius, L. *De justitia et jure*. Leuven, 1605.

Mansi, J. *Sacrorum conciliorum nova et amplissima collectio*. Florence, 1759–1798.

Marc, C., and F. X. Gestermann. *Institutiones morales alphonsianae*, 18th ed. Edited by J. Raus. Lyon: Vitte, 1927.

Mazzotta, N. *Theologia moralis*. Venice, 1760.

McFadden, C. *Medical Ethics*. Philadelphia: F. A. Davis Co., 1955.

Merkelbach, B. *Summa theologiae moralis*. Paris:Desclée, 1935.

Meyer, T. *Institutiones iuris naturalis*. Freiburg: Herder, 1900.

Molina, L. *De iustitia et iure*. Cologne, 1614.

———. *De justitia et jure*. Venice, 1611.

Noldin, H., and A. Schmitt. *Summa theologiae moralis*. 27th ed. Innsbruck: Rauch, 1940–41.

Paquin, J. *Morale et medécine*. Montreal: L'Immaculée-Conception, 1955.

Patuzzi, V. *Ethica Christiana sive theologia moralis.* Bassani, 1770.

Payen, G. *Déontologie medicale d'après droit natural, résumé.* Zikawei, China: Imprimerie de la Mission Catholique, 1928.

Pighi, J. *Cursus theologiae moralis.* Verona, 1901.

Pius XI. *Casti connubii.* December 31, 1930. In H. Denzinger, *Enchiridion symbolorum definitionum et declarationum de rebus fidei et morum.* Edited by J. Umberg. Freiburg: Herder, 1942.

Pius XII. "Address to the First International Congress on the Histopathology of the Nervous System." September 14, 1952. In *Discorsi e Radiomessaggi di Sua Santità Pio XII*, vol. 14, *March 2, 1952–March 1, 1953.* Vatican City: Typographia Polyglotta Vaticana, 1953.

Prümmer, D. *Manuale theologiae moralis.* Freiburg: Herder, 1933.

Rabanus Maurus. *Commentaria in libros machabaeorum.* Vol. 109 of *Patrologiae cursus completus, series latina.* Paris: Migne, 1844–1864.

Regatillo, E.F., and M. Zalba. *Theologiae moralis summa.* Madrid: Biblioteca de Autores Cristianos, 1953.

Reiffenstuel, A. *Theologia moralis.* Modena, 1740.

Riley, L. *The History, Nature and Use of Epikeia in Moral Theology.* Washington, D.C.: Catholic University of America Press, 1948), p. 137.

Rodrigo, L. *Praelectiones theologico-morales comillenses .* Santander: Sal Terrae, 1944.

Roncaglia, C. *Theologia moralis.* Lucca, 1730.

Salmanticenses. *Cursus theologiae moralis.* Lyon, 1879.

Sanchez, T. *Consilia seu opuscula moralia.* Lyon, 1681.

Sayrus, G. *Clavis regia casuum conscientae.* Venice, 1625.

Scavini, P. *Theologia moralis universa* (Turin: Marietti, 1865), II, n. 708.

Schuster, J. B. *Philosophia moralis.* Freiburg: Herder, 1950.

Sertillanges, R. P. *La philosophie morale de Thomas d'Aquin.* Paris: Aubier-Montaigne, 1946.

Somme theologique Saint Thomas D'Aquin. Paris: Desclée, 1934.

Soto, D. *De justitia et jure.* Lyon, 1582.

Sporer, P. *Theologica moralis.* Venice, 1766.

Suarez, F. *Opera omnia.* Edited by C. Berton. Paris, 1858.

Sullivan, C., and E. Campbell. "One Thousand Cesarean Sections in the Modern Era of Obstetrics." *Linacre Quarterly* (November 1955): 117–126.

Sullivan, J. *Catholic Teaching on the Morality of Euthanasia.* Washington, D.C.: University of America Press, 1949.

Tamburini, T. *Explicatio decalogi.* Venice, 1719.

Tanquerey, A. *Synopsis theologiae moralis et pastoralis.* Paris: Desclée & Socii, 1953.

Taylor, R. "Consent for Treatment." *Linacre Quarterly* 22.4 (November 1955): 131–135.

Tournely, H. *Theologica moralis.* Venice, 1756.

Ubach, J. *Theologia moralis.* Buenos Aires: Sociedad San Miguel, 1935.

Vander Heeren, A. "Suicide." In *The Catholic Encyclopedia,* Vol. 14. New York, Appleton Co., 1912.

Vermeersch, A. *Quaestiones de virtutibus religonis et pietatis.* Bruges: Bayaert, 1912.

————. *Theologiae moralis principia-responsa-consilia.* 3rd ed. Rome: Pontificia Universitas Gregoriana, 1945.

Vitoria, F. de. *Comentarios a la secunda secundae de Santo Tomas.* Salamanca, 1932–1952.

————. *De homicidio.* Lecture 10 in *Relectiones theologicae.* Lyon, 1587.

————. *De temperantia.* Lecture 9 in *Relectiones theologicae.* Lyon, 1587.

Vives y Tuto, J. *Compendium theologiae moralis,* 9th ed. Rome: Pustet, 1909.

Waffelaert, G. *De justitia.* Vol. 2 of *De virtutibus cardinalibus.* Bruges, 1886.

Index of Authors